HEALTH CARE ISSUES, COSTS AND ACCESS

MEDICARE PAYMENT POLICIES AND ISSUES

HEALTH CARE ISSUES, COSTS AND ACCESS

Additional books in this series can be found on Nova's website under the Series tab.

Additional E-books in this series can be found on Nova's website under the E-book tab.

HEALTH CARE ISSUES, COSTS AND ACCESS

MEDICARE PAYMENT POLICIES AND ISSUES

ALEXANDER D. HOFFMANN
EDITOR

Nova Science Publishers, Inc.
New York

LIBRARY OF CONGRESS CATALOGING-IN-PUBLICATION DATA

Medicare payment policies and issues / editor, Alexander D. Hoffmann.
p. ; cm. -- (Health care issues, costs, and access)
Includes bibliographical references and index.
ISBN 978-1-61122-896-0 (hardcover : alk. paper)
1. Medicare. I. Hoffmann, Alexander D. II. Series: Health care issues, costs, and access.
[DNLM: 1. Medicare--economics. 2. Fee Schedules--legislation & jurisprudence--United States. 3. Health Policy--United States. 4. Insurance, Health, Reimbursement--legislation & jurisprudence--United States. 5. Prospective Payment System--legislation & jurisprudence--United States. WT 31]
RA412.3.M439 2011
368.4'2600973--dc22

2010047027

Published by Nova Science Publishers, Inc. † New York

CONTENTS

PREFACE

Payment policies for certain medical services, such as physician services and the most durable medical equipment are based on fee schedules. This book provides an overview of Medicare payment rules by type of service, outlines current payment policies and summarizes the basic rules for program updates.

Chapter 1 - Medicare is a federal insurance program that pays for covered health services for most persons 65 years of age and older and for most permanently disabled individuals under the age of 65. Part A of the program, the Hospital Insurance program, covers hospital, post-hospital, and hospice services. Part B, the Supplementary Medical Insurance program, covers a broad range of complementary medical services including physician, laboratory, outpatient hospital services, and durable medical equipment. Part C provides private plan options for beneficiaries enrolled in both Parts A and B. Part D is an optional outpatient prescription drug program.

Medicare has established specific rules for payment of covered benefits. Some, such as physician services and most durable medical equipment, are based on fee schedules. Some payments are based, in part, on a provider's bid (an estimate of the cost of providing a service) relative to a benchmark (the maximum amount Medicare will pay). Bids and benchmarks are used to determine payments in Medicare Parts C and D. Payments for some items of durable medical equipment in specified locations are to be based on competitive bidding, starting in 2011. Many services, however, including inpatient and outpatient hospital care, are paid under different prospective payment systems (PPSs). In general, the program provides for annual updates to these payment amounts. The program also has rules regarding the amount of cost sharing, if any, which beneficiaries can be billed in excess of Medicare's recognized payment levels. Unlike other services, Medicare's outpatient prescription drug benefit can be obtained only through private plans. Further, while all Part D plans must meet certain minimum requirements, they differ in terms of benefit design, formulary drugs, and cost-sharing amounts.

Medicare payment policies and potential changes to these policies are of continuing interest to Congress. The Medicare program has been a major focus of deficit reduction legislation since 1980. With certain exceptions, reductions in program spending have been achieved largely through regulating payments to providers, primarily hospitals and physicians. The Balanced Budget Act of 1997 (P.L. 105-33, BBA) modified some existing payment policies, including changing underlying payment methodologies and updates to payment amounts. Subsequent legislation increased Medicare funding to mitigate the financial impact of some BBA provisions. The Medicare Prescription Drug, Improvement, and Modernization Act of 2003 (P.L. 108-173, MMA), too, modified payment methods and established payment increases for some providers. Most recently, the Tax Relief and Health Care Act of 2006 (P.L. 109-432, TRHCA); the Medicare, Medicaid, and SCHIP Extension Act of 2007 (P.L. 110-173, MMSEA); the Medicare Improvements for Patients and Providers Act of 2008 (P.L. 110-275, MIPPA); and the Patient Protection and Affordable Care Act of 2010 (P.L. 111-148), as modified by the Health Care and Education Reconciliation Act of 2010 (P.L. 111-152), have affected Medicare's payments.

This report provides an overview of Medicare payment rules by type of service, outlines current payment policies, and summarizes the basic rules for program updates. This report will be updated at least annually.

Chapter 2 - Each year since 2002, the statutory method for determining the annual updates to the Medicare physician fee schedule, known as the sustainable growth rate (SGR) system, has resulted in a reduction in the reimbursement rates (or a "negative update"). With the exception of 2002, when a 4.8% decrease was applied, Congress has passed a series of bills to override the reductions. The SGR system was established because of the concern that the Medicare fee schedule itself would not adequately constrain overall increases in spending for physicians' services. While the fee schedule limits the amount that Medicare will pay for each service, there are no limits on the volume or mix of services. The SGR system was intended to serve as a restraint on aggregate spending. If expenditures over a period are less than the cumulative spending target for the period, the update is increased. However, if spending exceeds the cumulative spending target over a certain period, future updates are reduced to bring spending back in line with the target.

In the first few years of the SGR system, the actual expenditures did not exceed the targets and the updates to the physician fee schedule were close to the Medicare economic index (MEI, a price index of inputs required to produce physician services) in the first two years (2.3% in 1998 and 1999, compared with a MEI of 2.2% in 1998 and 2.3% in 1999). For the next two years, in 2000 and 2001, the actual physician fee schedule update was more than twice the MEI for those years (5.5% update vs. MEI of 2.4% in 2000, 5.0% update vs. MEI of 2.1% in 2001). However, beginning in 2002, the actual expenditure exceeded allowed targets and the discrepancy has grown with each year, resulting in a series of ever-larger cuts under the formula.

Some criticisms of the SGR system point to purported flaws in the technical details behind the formula, while others have just expressed displeasure with the resultant outcome. Although modifications have been proposed to replace the SGR system, no proposal has garnered sufficient support and almost all proposals would be expensive to implement compared against the current baseline, which necessarily assumes that significant cuts to the fee schedule will occur.

Legislative activity in the current session of Congress includes several bills. The FY2010 Defense Appropriations Act delayed the implementation of the reductions for two months, through February 28, 2010. The Statutory Pay-As-You-Go Act of 2010 (P.L. 111-139) exempts the amount it would cost to freeze payments for five years from PAYGO rules. H.R. 4691, which became law on March 2, 2010, delayed the payment cuts through March 31, 2010. On April 15, the Senate passed an amended version of H.R. 4851 that extended the payment cut delay through May 31, 2010. The House passed the amended bill, and the President signed P.L. 111-157 into law that day. On June 25, 2010, several weeks after the expiration of the extension created by the Continuing Extension Act, an amended version of H.R. 3962 was signed into law that increases fee schedule payments 2.2% retroactive to June 1 and continuing through November 30, 2010.

Chapter 3 - Medicare's physician fees may not always reflect efficiencies that occur when a physician performs multiple services for the same patient on the same day, and some resources required for these services do not need to be duplicated. In response to a request from Congress, GAO examined (1) the Centers for Medicare & Medicaid Services' (CMS) efforts to set appropriate fees for services furnished together and (2) additional opportunities for CMS to avoid excessive payments when services are furnished together. GAO examined relevant policies, laws, and regulations; interviewed CMS officials and others; and analyzed claims data to identify opportunities for further savings.

Chapter 4 - According to the 2009 Medicare Trustees report, total Medicare expenditures were $468 billion dollars in 2008 for 45 million beneficiaries. The Office of the Actuary projects overall Medicare spending to reach $507.1 billion for 2009. Because of a number of factors, such as advances in health care delivery and technology, an aging population, and overall increases in medical costs, spending on Medicare services is expected to grow more quickly than spending in the U.S. economy. As expenditures continue to rise in the nation's largest health insurance program, efforts to preserve the integrity of the program receive increased attention from policy makers.

Chapter 5 - Recovery Audit Contractors, or RACs, are private organizations that contract with the Centers for Medicare and Medicaid Services (CMS) to identify and collect improper payments made in Medicare's fee-for-service (FFS) program. CMS projects improper FFS payments to amount to approximately $10.4 billion or 3.6% of all paid Medicare claims in 2008. Congress originally required the Secretary of the Department of Health and Human Services to conduct a three-year demonstration program using RACs in the Medicare Prescription Drug, Improvement, and Modernization Act of 2003 (MMA, P.L. 108-173). In December 2006, Congress passed the Tax Relief and Health Care Act of 2006 (TRHCA, P.L. 109-432), which made the program permanent and mandated the expansion of RACs nationwide by 2010. CMS began the national rollout of the permanent program in 19 states in March 2009.

In: Medicare Payment Policies and Issues
Editors: Alexander D. Hoffmann
ISBN: 978-1-61122-896-0

Chapter 1

MEDICARE PAYMENT POLICIES

Paulette C. Morgan, Patricia A. Davis, Barbara English, Jim Hahn, Mark Newsom, Julie Stone and Sibyl Tilson

SUMMARY

Medicare is a federal insurance program that pays for covered health services for most persons 65 years of age and older and for most permanently disabled individuals under the age of 65. Part A of the program, the Hospital Insurance program, covers hospital, post-hospital, and hospice services. Part B, the Supplementary Medical Insurance program, covers a broad range of complementary medical services including physician, laboratory, outpatient hospital services, and durable medical equipment. Part C provides private plan options for beneficiaries enrolled in both Parts A and B. Part D is an optional outpatient prescription drug program.

Medicare has established specific rules for payment of covered benefits. Some, such as physician services and most durable medical equipment, are based on fee schedules. Some payments are based, in part, on a provider's bid (an estimate of the cost of providing a service) relative to a benchmark (the maximum amount Medicare will pay). Bids and benchmarks are used to determine payments in Medicare Parts C and D. Payments for some items of durable medical equipment in specified locations are to be based on competitive bidding, starting in 2011. Many services, however, including inpatient and outpatient hospital care, are paid under different prospective payment systems (PPSs). In general, the program provides for annual updates to these payment amounts. The program also has rules regarding the amount of cost sharing, if any, which beneficiaries can be billed in excess of Medicare's recognized payment levels. Unlike other services, Medicare's outpatient prescription drug benefit can be obtained only through private plans. Further, while all Part D plans must meet certain minimum requirements, they differ in terms of benefit design, formulary drugs, and cost-sharing amounts.

Medicare payment policies and potential changes to these policies are of continuing interest to Congress. The Medicare program has been a major focus of deficit reduction legislation since 1980. With certain exceptions, reductions in program spending have been achieved largely through regulating payments to providers, primarily hospitals and physicians. The Balanced Budget Act of 1997 (P.L. 105-33, BBA) modified some existing payment policies, including changing underlying payment methodologies and updates to payment amounts. Subsequent legislation increased Medicare funding to mitigate the financial impact of some BBA provisions. The Medicare Prescription Drug, Improvement, and Modernization Act of 2003 (P.L. 108-173, MMA), too, modified payment methods and established payment increases for some providers. Most recently, the Tax Relief and Health Care Act of 2006 (P.L. 109-432, TRHCA); the Medicare, Medicaid, and SCHIP Extension Act of 2007 (P.L. 110-173, MMSEA); the Medicare Improvements for Patients and Providers Act of 2008 (P.L. 110-275, MIPPA); and the Patient Protection and Affordable Care Act of 2010 (P.L. 111-148), as modified by the Health Care and Education Reconciliation Act of 2010 (P.L. 111-152), have affected Medicare's payments.

This report provides an overview of Medicare payment rules by type of service, outlines current payment policies, and summarizes the basic rules for program updates. This report will be updated at least annually.

Introduction

Medicare is a federal insurance program that pays for covered health services for most persons 65 years of age and older and for most permanently disabled individuals under the age of 65. Part A of the program, the Hospital Insurance program, covers hospital services, up to 100 days of post- hospital skilled nursing facility services, post-institutional home health visits, and hospice services. Part B, the Supplementary Medical Insurance program, covers a broad range of medical services including physician services,[1] laboratory services, durable medical equipment, and outpatient hospital services. Part B also covers some home health visits. Part C (also known as Medicare Advantage, or MA) provides private plan options, such as managed care, for beneficiaries who are enrolled in both Parts A and B. Part D provides optional outpatient prescription drug coverage.

MEDICARE PAYMENT PRINCIPLES

In general, the total payment received by a provider for covered services provided to a Medicare beneficiary is composed of two parts: a program payment from Medicare plus any beneficiary cost-sharing that is required.[2] (The required beneficiary out-of-pocket payment may be paid by other insurance, if any.)[3] Medicare has established specific rules governing its program payments for all covered services as well as for beneficiary cost sharing as described below.

Medicare Payment Rules

Medicare has established specific rules governing payment for covered services For example, the program pays for most acute inpatient and outpatient hospital services, skilled nursing facility services, and home health care under a prospective payment system (PPS) established for the particular service; under PPS, a predetermined rate is paid for each unit of service such as a hospital discharge or payment classification group. Payments for physician services, clinical laboratory services, and certain durable medical equipment covered under Part B are made on the basis of fee schedules.[4] Certain other services are paid on the basis of reasonable costs or reasonable charges. In general, the program provides for annual updates of the program payments to reflect inflation and other factors. In some cases, these updates are linked to the consumer price index for all urban consumers (CPI-U) or to a provider-specific market basket (MB) index which measures the change in the price of goods and services purchased by the provider to produce a unit of output. However, updates to the physician fee schedule are determined by a statutory formula, known as the sustainable growth rate (SGR) system, which links annual updates to how cumulative actual expenditures compare with a cumulative expenditures target.[5]

Beneficiary Out-of-Pocket Payments

There are two aspects of beneficiary payments to providers: required cost-sharing amounts (either coinsurance, copayments, or deductibles) and the amounts that beneficiaries may be billed over and above Medicare's recognized payment amounts for certain services. For Part A, coinsurance and deductible amounts are established annually; these payments include deductibles and coinsurance for hospital services, coinsurance for skilled nursing facilities (SNFs), no cost sharing for home health services, and nominal cost sharing for hospice care.[6] For Part B, beneficiaries are generally responsible for premiums, which range from $110.50 to $353.60 in 2010, depending on the beneficiary's income, a $155 deductible in 2010 (updated annually by the increase in the Part B premium), and a coinsurance payment of 20% of the established Medicare payment amounts.[7] For Part C, cost sharing is determined by the private plans. Through 2005, the total of premiums[8] for *basic* Medicare benefits and cost sharing (deductibles, coinsurance, and co-payments) charged to a Part C enrollee could not exceed actuarially determined levels of cost sharing for those same benefits under original Medicare. This meant that plans could not charge a premium for Medicare-covered benefits without reducing cost-sharing amounts. Beginning in 2006, the constraint on a plan's ability to charge a premium for *basic* Medicare benefits was lifted. The bidding mechanism established by the MMA allows plans to charge a premium to cover *basic* Medicare benefits if the costs to the plan exceed the maximum amount CMS will pay for Medicare-covered benefits. The MMA eliminated the explicit inverse relationship between cost sharing for *basic* Medicare benefits and a premium for *basic* Medicare benefits. Aggregate enrollee cost sharing under Part C is now only constrained by the actuarial value of cost sharing under original Medicare.[9] However, also beginning in 2006, the Secretary has expanded authority to negotiate or reject a bid from a managed care organization in order to ensure that the bid reasonably reflects the plan's revenue requirements. Part D cost sharing includes a deductible, co- payments, and catastrophic limits on out-of-pocket spending.

For most services, there are rules on amounts beneficiaries may be billed over and above Medicare's recognized payment amounts. Under Part A, providers agree to accept Medicare's payment as payment in full and cannot bill beneficiaries amounts in excess of the coinsurance and deductibles. Under Part B, providers and practitioners are subject to limits on the amounts they can bill beneficiaries for covered services depending on their participation status in the Medicare program. A *participating physician* agrees to accept the approved fee schedule amount as payment in full (assignment) for all services delivered to Medicare beneficiaries, of which 80% is paid by the Medicare program and the beneficiary is responsible for the 20% coinsurance plus any unmet deductible. Physicians who do not agree to accept assignment on all Medicare claims in a given year are referred to as *nonparticipating physicians*. Nonparticipating physicians may or may not accept assignment for a given service. If they do not, they may charge beneficiaries more than the fee schedule amount on nonassigned claims; for physicians, these *balance billing* charges are subject to certain limits.

Assignment is mandatory for some providers, such as nurse practitioners, physician assistants, and clinical laboratories; these providers can only bill the beneficiary the 20% coinsurance and any unmet deductible. For other Part B services, such as durable medical equipment, assignment is optional; providers may bill beneficiaries for amounts above Medicare's recognized payment level and may do so without limit.

Recent Congressional Actions with Respect to Program Payments

Because of its rapid growth, both in terms of aggregate dollars and as a share of the federal budget, the Medicare program has been a major focus of congressional deficit reduction legislation, as outlined below. With a few exceptions, savings in program spending have been achieved largely through reductions in the updates to provider payments, primarily hospitals, physicians, and MA plans. However, even when payments are frozen (as has been the case with payments to acute care hospitals, inpatient rehabilitation facilities, long term care hospitals, and with the physician fee schedule), Medicare spending continues to increase each year.

Most recently the Patient Protection and Affordable Care Act (P.L. 111-148, PPACA), as amended, is estimated to achieve substantial program savings through permanent reductions in the maximum amount paid to MA plans, and reductions in the annual updates to Medicare's feefor-service (FFS) providers (other than physicians' services). The anticipated savings from FFS providers is substantially due to the application of a productivity adjustment. (Productivity, in general, is a measure of output produced relative to the amount of work required to produce it.[10]) PPACAs update reductions mark a departure from most previous legislative actions to reduce Medicare program spending, first, because it is a permanent adjustment to (non-physician) payment updates,[11] and second, because, in general, it specifies that the adjustment allows for negative payment updates and as such, payment rates for a year may be less than for a preceding year. Once the estimates of savings are known, Congress may wish to revisit this issue whether rates are much higher or much lower than originally estimated. As in the case of physician payment updates, it is unclear whether Congress will allow providers to be paid less under this new provision. As the Medicare Trustees emphasized in the 2010 Annual Report, "the very favorable financial outcomes that would be experienced if the productivity adjustments can be sustained in the long range" are highly dependent on the actual implementation of the provisions, although the trustees "recognize the great uncertainty associated with achieving this outcome."[12]

RECENT LEGISLATIVE HISTORY

The Balanced Budget Act of 1997 (P.L. 105-33, BBA 97) achieved significant savings to the Medicare program by slowing the rate of growth in payments to providers and by enacting structural changes to the program.[13] A number of health care provider groups stated that actual Medicare benefit payment reductions resulting from BBA were larger than were intended, leading to facility closings and other limits on beneficiary access to care. In November 1999, Congress passed a package of funding increases to mitigate the impact of some BBA 97 provisions on providers. This measure, the Medicare, Medicaid, and SCHIP Balanced Budget Refinement Act of 1999 (BBRA), is part of a larger measure known as the Consolidated Appropriations Act for 2000 (P.L. 106-113).[14] Further adjustments were made by the Medicare, Medicaid, and SCHIP Benefits Improvement and Protection Act (BIPA), part of the larger Consolidated Appropriations Act, 2001 (P.L. 106-554).[15] In addition to increasing Medicare payment rates, the subsequent legislation mandated the development or refinement of PPSs for different Medicare covered services. The Medicare Prescription Drug, Improvement, and Modernization Act of 2003 (P.L. 108-173, MMA)[16] contained a major benefit expansion in adding prescription drug coverage; Congress included a number of provisions that affected payments to providers and changed administrative and contracting procedures. Further modifications were made to Medicare payments in the Deficit Reduction Act of 2005 (P.L. 109-171, DRA)[17]; the Tax Relief and Health Care Act of 2006 (P.L. 109-432, TRHCA); the Medicare, Medicaid, and SCHIP Extension Act of 2007 (P.L. 110-173, MMSEA)[18]; and the Medicare Improvements for Patients and Providers Act of 2008 (P.L. 110-275, MIPPA)[19]; and the Patient Protection and Affordable Care Act (P.L. 111- 148, PPACA) as modified by the Health Care and Education Reconciliation Act (P.L. 111-152, HCERA).[20]

This report provides a guide to Medicare payment rules by type of benefit. It includes a summary of current payment policies and basic rules for updating payment amounts. It is updated to reflect the most recent legislative changes to the program and payment updates available through July 2010.

Medicare Payment Policies

Part A

Table 1. Inpatient Prospective Payment System (IPPS) for Short-term, General Hospitals

Provider/service	General payment policy	General update policy	Recent update
Operating PPS for inpatient services provided by acute hospitals (Operating IPPS)	Medicare pays acute care hospitals using a prospectively determined payment for each discharge. A hospital's payment for its operating costs is calculated using a national standardized amount adjusted by a wage index associated with the area where the hospital is located or where it has been reclassified. Payment also depends on the relative resource use associated with the diagnosis related group (DRG) to which the patient is assigned. A new Medicare Severity DRG (MS-DRG) patient classification system is being phased in starting in FY2008. Medicare pays additional	After accounting for certain budget neutrality adjustments, IPPS payment rates are increased annually by an update factor that is determined, in part, by the projected increase in the hospital market basket (MB) index. This is a fixed price index that measures the change in the price of goods and services purchased by hospitals to create one unit of output. The update for operating IPPS is established by statute. Under DRA, hospitals that do not submit required quality data in FY2007 and each subsequent year will have the applicable MB percentage reduced by two percentage points. Any MB	**For FY2009**, hospitals that submitted the required quality data received the full MB increase of 3.6%. The national standardized amount for these hospitals was 5,128.41. Hospitals that did not submit the quality data received a reduced update of 1.6%. The national standardized amount for these hospitals was $5,029.40. **For FY2010,** effective for discharges after April 1, 2010, hospitals that submitted the required quality data receive an update of 1.85%. The national standardized amount for these hospitals is $5,212.02.

Table 1. (Continued)

Provider/service	General payment policy	General update policy	Recent update
	amounts for cases with extra-ordinary costs (outliers); indirect medical education (IME) (see below); and for hospitals serving a disproportionate share (DSH) of low-income patients (see below). IME and DSH payments are made through adjustments within IPPS so that hospitals receive more money for each Medicare discharge. Additional payments may be made for cases that involve qualified new technologies that have been approved for special add-on payments. Hospitals in Hawaii and Alaska receive a cost-of-living adjustment (COLA). Certain services are reimbursed outside of IPPS.	reduction does not apply when computing the applicable percentage increase in subsequent years. In its FY2008 rule, CMS established prospective budget neutrality adjustments of -1.2% in FY2008, -1.8% in FY2009 and -1.8% in FY2010 because of anticipated increases in measured severity of illness because of coding changes or documentation improvements (coding creep) associated with the new MS-DRGs. P.L. 110-90 reduced the adjustment to 0.6% in FY2008 and 0.9% in FY2009, but permits offsets to IPPS rate increases in FY2010, FY2011, and FY2012 to account for coding creep increases in FY2008 and FY2009 above these amounts. The law did not address the scheduled adjustment of an additional 1.8% decrease in FY2010. PPACA established a schedule of annual	Hospitals that did not submit the quality data receive a reduced update of -0.15%. The national standardized amount for these hospitals is $5,111.64.

Table 1. (Continued)

Provider/service	General payment policy	General update policy	Recent update
		reductions in the update for FY2009 through FY2019. The reduction in the FY2010 IPPS update of 0.25 percentage points became effective for discharges starting April 1, 2010. The annual update will include a productivity adjustment starting October 1, 2011. The PPACA update reductions may result in a negative update for that year.	
Capital IPPS for short-term general hospitals (Capital IPPS)	Medicare's capital IPPS is structured similarly to its operating IPPS for short-term general hospitals. A hospital's capital payment is based on a prospectively determined federal payment rate, depends on the DRG to which the patient is assigned, and is adjusted by a hospital's geographic adjustment factor (which is calculated from the hospital's wage index data). Capital IPPS includes an IME and DSH adjustment (see below).	Updates to the capital IPPS are not established in statute. Capital rates are updated annually by the Centers for Medicare and Medicaid (CMS) according to a framework which considers changes in the prices associated with capital-related costs as measured by the capital input price index (CIPI) and other policy factors, including changes in case mix intensity, errors in previous CIPI forecasts, DRG recalibration, and DRG	The capital IPPS update for FY2009 was 0.9%, which reflects an estimated increase in the CIPI and a downward adjustment of 0.5% to account for DRG reclassification and recalibration. After applying other adjustments, the FY2009 federal capital rate was $424.17, a -0.51% change from the prior year. The capital IPS update for FY2010 is 1.4% attributable to the current forecast of the CIPI

Table 1. (Continued)

Provider/service	General payment policy	General update policy	Recent update
	Starting in FY2008, the IME adjustment will be phased out over a 3-year period. Additional payments are made for outliers (cases with significantly higher costs above a certain threshold). Certain hospitals may also qualify for additional payments under an exceptions process. A new hospital is paid 85% of its allowable Medicare inpatient hospital capital-related costs for its first two years of operation.	reclassification. Other adjustments include those that implement budget neutrality with respect to recalibration of DRGs, documentation and coding changes resulting from the switch to MS-DRGs that do not reflect real changes in patient severity of illness, real outlier payments, changes in the geographic adjustment factor, and exception payments.	available when the final rule was published. After adjustments, the FY2010 capital federal rates is $429.56 for discharges starting April 1, 2010.
Disproportionate share hospital (DSH) adjustment	Approximately 2,800 hospitals receive the additional payments for each Medicare discharge based on a formula which incorporates the number of patient days provided to low-income Medicare beneficiaries (those who receive Supplemental Security Income (SSI)) and Medicaid recipients. A few urban hospitals, known as "Pickle Hospitals," receive DSH	No specific update. The amount of DSH spending in any year is open-ended and varies by the number of Medicare discharges as well as the type of patient seen in any given hospital.	CBO estimates DSH spending (in both operating and capital IPPS) at $9.48 billion in FY2008 and $10.1 billion in FY2009 in its March 2009 baseline.

Table 1. (Continued)

Provider/service	General payment policy	General update policy	Recent update
	payments under an alternative formula that considers the proportion of a hospital's patient care revenues that are received from state and local indigent care funds. The percentage add-on for which a hospital will qualify varies according to the hospital's bed size or urban or rural location. The DSH adjustment for most categories of hospitals is capped at 12%. Urban hospitals with more than 100 beds, rural hospitals with more than 500 beds, Medicare dependent hospitals (MDHs, see below), and rural referral centers (RRC, see below) are exempt from the 12% DSH adjustment cap.		
Indirect Medical Education (IME) adjustment	The indirect medical education (IME) adjustment is one of two types of payments to teaching hospitals for graduate medical education (GME) costs (see also direct GME below). Medicare	The IME adjustment is not subject to an annual update. BBA 97 reduced the IME adjustment in operating IPPS from a 7.7% increase for each 10% increase in a hospital's ratio of interns to	No specific update. The amount spent on IME depends in part on the number of Medicare discharges in teaching hospitals in any given year. CBO estimates the IME

Table 1. (Continued)

Provider/service	General payment policy	General update policy	Recent update
	increases both its operating and capital IPPS payments to teaching hospitals; different measures of teaching intensity are used in the operating and capital IPPS. For both IPPS payments, however, the number of medical residents who can be counted for the IME adjustment is capped, based on the number of medical residents as of December 31, 1996. As established by BBA 97, teaching hospitals also receive IME payments for their Medicare Part C discharges. (See also Medicare Part C below.)	beds (IRB), a measure of teaching intensity in operating IPPS; by FY2001, the IME adjustment was to be 5.5%. However, the scheduled decreases were delayed by subsequent legislation. As established by MMA, the IME adjustment was set at 5.5% in FY2008 and subsequently.	payments (for both capital and operating IPPS) to be about $5.7 billion in FY2008 and $6.1 billion in FY2009 in its March 2009 baseline.
Direct graduate medical education (direct GME) payments	Direct GME costs are excluded from IPPS and paid outside of the DRG payment on the basis of updated hospital-specific costs per resident amount (PRA), the number of weighted full- time equivalent (FTE) residents, and Medicare's share of total patient days in the hospital (including	In general, direct GME payments are updated by the increase in the consumer price index for all urban consumers (CPI-U). As established by BBRA and sub-sequently amended, however, the update amount that any hospital receives depends upon the relationship of its PRA to the	Hospitals below 140% of the national average from FY2004-FY2013 receive an update of CPI-U. Hospitals above 140% of the national average for that time period will receive no update. CBO estimates direct GME payments of $3.2 billion in **FY2008** and in **FY2009** in

Table 1. (Continued)

Provider/service	General payment policy	General update policy	Recent update
	those days attributed to Medicare manged care enrollees). There is a hospital- specific cap on the number of residents in the hospital for direct GME payments. Also, the hospital's FTE count is based on a three-year rolling average; a specific resident may count as half of a FTE, depending on the number of years spent as a resident and the length of the initial training associated with the specialty. Certain combined primary care residency programs receive special recognition in this count. In certain circumstances, irect GME payments can be made to nonhospital providers.	national average PRA. Hospitals with PRAs below the floor (85% of the locality-adjusted, updated, and weighted national PRA) are raised to the floor amount. Teaching hospitals with PRAs above the ceiling amount (140% of the national average, adjusted for geographic location) will receive a lower update than other hospitals (CPI-U minus two percentage points) for FY2003-FY2013. Hospitals that have PRAs between the floor and ceiling receive the CPI-U as an update amount.	its March 2009 baseline.

Table 2. Hospitals Receiving Special Consideration Under Medicare's IPPS

Provider/service	General payment policy	General update policy	Recent update
Sole Community Hospitals (SCHs)— facilities located in geographically isolated areas and deemed to be the sole provider of inpatient acute care hospital services in a geographic area based on distance, travel time, severe weather condi-tions, and/or mar-ket share as criteria set forth in regulation (42 CFR 412.92).	An SCH receives the higher of the following payment rates as the basis of reimbursement: the current IPPS base payment rate, or its hospital-specific per-discharge costs from either FY1982, 1987, or 1996, updated to the current year. Under MIPPA, for cost reporting periods beginning on or after January 1, 2009, an SCH will be able to elect payment based on its FY2006 hospital-specific payment amount per discharge. This amount will be increased by the annual update starting for discharges on or after January 1, 2009. An SCH may receive additional payments if the hospital experiences a decrease of more than 5% in its total inpatient cases due to circumstances beyond its control. An SCH receives special consideration for reclassification into a different area. Starting for services on January 1, 2006, CMS increased outpatient prospective payment system (OPPS) payments to rural SCHs by an additional 7.1%.	Target amounts for SCHs are updated by an "appli-cable percentage increase" which is specified by statute and is often comparable to the IPPS update. (See description for IPPS hospitals).	**For FY2009,** hospitals that submitted the required quality data received the full MB increase of 3.6%. Hospitals that did not submit the quality data received a reduced update of 1.6%. **For FY2010**, starting for discharges on April 1, 2010, hospitals that submitted the required quality data receive an update of 1.85%. Hospitals that did not submit the quality data receive a reduced update of -0.15%.
Medicare dependent hospitals (MDHs)— small rural hospitals with a high pro-portion of patients who are Medicare beneficiaries	BBA 97 reinstated and extended the MDH classification, starting on October 1, 1997, and extending to October 1, 2001. The sunset date for the MDH classification was subsequently extended to September 30, 2011 by DRA. Until	Target amounts for MDHs are updated by an "applicable percentage increase" which is specified by	For FY1996 and thereafter, the update for MDHs is the same as for all IPPS hospitals. These updates are also used to increase the

Table 2. (Continued)

Provider/service	General payment policy	General update policy	Recent update
(have at least 60% of acute inpatient days or discharges attributable to Medicare in FY1987 or in two of the three most recently audited cost reporting periods). As specified in regulation (42 CFR 412.108), they cannot be an SCH and must Provider/service have 100 or fewer beds.	October 1, 2006, an MDH was paid the federal rate plus 50% of the amount that the rate is exceeded by the hospital's target amount based on either its updated FY1982 or FY1987 cost per discharge. DRA provided that an MDH would be able to elect payments based on using a percentage of its FY2002 hospital-specific cost starting October 1, 2006. An MDH's payments would be based on 75% of the adjusted hospital-specific cost starting for discharges on October 1, 2006. DRA also excluded MDHs from the 12% DSH adjustment cap for discharges starting October 1, 2006. An MDH may receive additional payments if its inpatient cases decline more than 5% due to General payment policy circumstances beyond its control.	statute and is often comparable to the IPPS update.	hospital-specific rate applicable to an MDH. For **FY2009,** hospitals that submitted the required quality data received the full MB increase of 3.6%. Hospitals that did not submit the quality data received a reduced update of 1.6% For **FY2010**, starting for discharges on April 1, 2010, hospitals that submitted the required quality data receive an update of 1.85%. Hospitals that did not submit the quality data receive a reduced update of -0.15%.
Rural Referral Centers (RRCs)—relatively large hospitals, generally in rural areas, that provide a broad array of services and treat patients from a wide geographic area as established by specific criteria set forth in regulation. (42 CFR 412.96).	RRCs payments are based on the IPPS for short-term general hospitals. RRCs are exempt from the 12% DSH adjustment cap. Also, RRCs receive preferential consideration for reclassification to a different area.	General update policy RRCs receive the operating and capital IPPS updates specified for short-term general hospitals.	Recent update See updates specified for operating and capital IPPS for short-term general hospitals.

Table 3. IPPS-Exempt Hospitals and Distinct Part Units

Provider/service	General payment policy	General update policy	Recent update
Inpatient Rehabilitation Facilities (IRFs)—freestanding hospitals and hospital-based distinct part units that treat a percentage of patients with a defined set of conditions and meet certain established conditions of participation. As established by MMSEA, starting July 1, 2007, the IRF compliance threshold (which determines whether a facility is an IRF or an acute care hospital) is set at 60%; comorbidities are included as qualifying conditions. To be paid as an IRF, an entity must have	As of January 1, 2002, Medicare's payments to a rehabilitation facility are based on a fully implemented IRF-PPS and 100% of the federal rate which is a fixed amount per discharge. This PPS encompasses both capital and operating payments to IRFs, but does not cover the costs of approved educational programs, bad debt expenses, or blood clotting factors, which are paid for separately. The IRF-PPS payment for any Medicare discharge will vary depending on the patient's impairment level, functional status, comorbidity conditions, and age. These factors determine which of the 87 Case Mix Groups (CMGs) is assigned to the inpatient stay. Within each of these CMGs, patients are further assigned to one of four tiers based on any comorbidities they may have. Five other	Starting in FY2006, the IRF-PPS update is based on the MB reflecting 2002 cost structures from rehabilitation, psychiatric, and long-term care hospitals (RPL-MB). The RLP-MBincludes an update estimate for capital as well as operating costs. MMSEA establishes the IRF update factor at 0% in FY2008 and FY2009, starting for discharges on April 1, 2008. PPACA established a schedule of annual reductions in the update for FY2009 through FY2019. The reduction in the FY2010 update of 0.25 percentage points became effective for discharges starting April 1, 2010. The annual update will include a productivity adjustment starting October 1, 2011. The PPACA update reductions may result in a negative update for that year.	In the FY2008 IRF rule CMS established the update for **FY2008** as 3.2% and the base federal rate as $13,451. However, in December 2007, MMSEA established the IRF update factor at 0% in FY2008 and FY2009 starting for discharges on April 1, 2008. The federal base rate was set at $12,981 starting April 1, 2008, and remained that amount through FY2009. The **FY2010** IRF-PPS update was 2.5% before the enactment of PPACA which imposed a 0.25 percentage point reduction on the FY2010 update (to 2.25%) for discharges starting April

Table 3. (Continued)

Provider/service	General payment policy	General update policy	Recent update
60% of its inpatients with one of 13 conditions including stroke, spinal cord injury, brain injury, neurological disorder, burns, and certain arthritis related conditions.	CMGs are used for patients discharged before the fourth day (short stay outliers) and for those who die in the facility. Generally, IRF payments are reduced or increased for certain case level adjustments, such as early transfers, short-stay outliers, patients who die before transfer, and high cost outliers. Payments also depend upon facility-specific adjustments to accommodate for variations in area wages, percentage of low income patients (LIP) served by the hospital (a DSH adjustment), and rural location (rural IRFs receive increased payments, about 19% more than urban IRFs.) Starting in FY2006, an IME adjustment is included; IRFs in Alaska and Hawaii do not receive a COLA adjustment. The IRF-PPS is not required to be budget neutral; total payments can exceed the amount that would have		1, 2010. Starting then, the base federal rate for IRFs is $13,627.

Table 3. (Continued)

Provider/service	General payment policy	General update policy	Recent update
	been paid if this PPS had not been implemented.		
Long-Term Care Hospitals and satellites or onsite providers (LTCHs)—acute general hospitals that are excluded from IPPS with a Medicare inpatient average length of stay (ALOS) greater than 25 days.	Effective October 1, 2002, LTCHs are paid on a discharge basis under a DRG-based PPS, subject to a five-year transition period. The LTCH-PPS encompasses payments for both operating and capital-related costs of inpatient care but does not cover the costs of approved educational programs, bad debt expenses, or blood clotting factors which are paid for separately. The LTCH-PPS payment for any Medicare discharge will vary depending on the patient's assignment into a Medicare severity- LTC-DRG. LT-DRGs are based on reweighted IPPS MS-DRGs. Payments for specific patients may be increased or reduced because of case-level adjustments, such as short stay cases, interrupted stay cases, readmitted cases from co-located	The LTCH update is not specified in statue. CMS has established a policy to update the LTCH rates based on the most recent estimate of the rehabili-tation, psychiatric, and long-term care (RPL) market basket adjusted to account for improved coding practices. CMS changed the effective date of the annual update from October 1 to July 1 of each year, starting July 2003. MMSEA established a three-year moratorium period during which the Secretary will not be able to apply certain payment policies, including payments for short stay outliers or the one-time adjustment to LTCH prospective payments to ensure budget neutrality. In the RY2009 final rule, CMS changed the effective date of the annual update back to	The **RY2009** (from July 1, 2008 through September 30, 2009) federal payment rate was $39,114.36. This increase was based on a MB estimate of 3.5% adjusted by 0.9% to account for the increase in case-mix in the prior period that resulted from changes in coding practices. The effective increase in the federal payment rate was 2.6%. In RY2010, (starting October 1, 2010) the LTCH federal payment rate was increased by 2.0% which reflects a 2.5% MB increase adjusted for case-mix changes attributed to

Table 3. (Continued)

Provider/service	General payment policy	General update policy	Recent update
	providers and high costs outliers. Payments also depend upon facility-specific adjustments such as variations in area wages and include a COLA for hospitals in Alaska and Hawaii. No adjust-ments are made for the percentage of low income patients served by the hospital (DSH), rural location, or IME. The LTCH-PPS is requi-red to be budget neutral; total payments must equal the amount that would have been paid if PPS had not been implemented.	October 1, beginning October 1, 2009. In order to implement the change, RY2009 will be a 15-month rate year, from July 1, 2008, through September 30, 2009. PPACA established a schedule of annual reductions in the update for RY2009 through RY2019. The reduction in the RY2010 update of 0.25 percentage points became effective for discharges starting April 1, 2010. The update will include a productivity adjustment starting October 1, 2011. The PPACA update reductions may result in a negative update for that year.	documentation and coding improvements. For discharges starting April 1, 2010, the update will be reduced by 0.25 percentage points; the LTCH federal payment rate is set at $39,794.95 for discharges starting on that date until September 30, 2010.
Psychiatric hospitals and distinct part units —include those primarily engaged in providing, by or under the supervision of a psychiatrist,	Starting January 1, 2005, Medicare pays for services provided in inpatient psychiatric facilities (IPF) using a per-diem based PPS. Established with a three-year transition period, the IPF-PPS incorporates patient-level	The IPF update is not specified in statue. CMS has established a policy to update the per diem rates based on the most recent estimate of the rehabilitation, psychiatric, and long-term care market basket (RPL-MB) The	The RPL-MB update for RY2010 was 2.1% After applying a wage index budget neutrality factor of 1.0009, the federal base payment is $651.76 per day. The

Table 3. (Continued)

Provider/service	General payment policy	General update policy	Recent update
psychiatric services for the diagnosis and treatment of people with mental illness.	adjustments for specified DRGs, selected comorbidies, and in certain cases, age of the patient. Facility-level adjustments for relative wages, teaching status and rural location are also included. IPFs in Hawaii and Alaska will receive a COLA adjustment. Medicare per diem payments are higher in the earlier days of the psychiatric stay. Also, the per diem payment for the first day of each stay is 12% higher in IFFs with qualifying (full-service) emergency departments than in other IPFs. An outlier policy for high-cost cases is included. Patients who are discharged from an IPF and return within three days are considered readmissions of the same case. IPFs also receive an additional payment for each eletroconvulsive Therapy treatment furnished to a patient. Finally, under the stop-loss provision, during the three-year	IPF-PPS payments must be projected to equal the amount of total payments that would have been made under the prior payment system. The initial calculation of the per diem payment included a 17.46% reduction to account for standardization to projected TEFRA (the prior payment system) payments, a 2% reduction to account for outlier payments, a 0.39% reduction to account for the stop-loss provision and a 2.66% reduction to account for a behavioral offset (to reflect changing utilization under the new payment system). PPACA established a schedule of annual reductions in the update starting RY2011 through RY2020. The reduction in the RY2011 IPF update of 0.25 percentage points effective July 1, 2010. The update will include a productivity	RPL-MB update for RY2011 is 2.4%,,reduced by the PPACA offset of 0.25 percentage points and a wage index budget neutrality offset of 0.9999. The federal base payment is $665.71 per day.

Table 3. (Continued)

Provider/service	General payment policy	General update policy	Recent update
	transition period ending in 2008, an IPF is guaranteed at least 70% of the aggregate payments that would have been made under the prior payment system.	adjustment starting July 1, 2012. The PPACA update reductions may result in a negative update for that year.	
Children's and cancer hospitals: ***Children's hospitals*** are those engaged in furnishing services to inpatients who are predominan-tly individuals under the age of 18. **Cancer hospitals** are generally recognized by the National Cancer Institute as either a comprehen-sive or clinical cancer research center; are primarily organized for the treatment of and research on cancer (not as a	Children's and cancer hospitals are paid on a reasonable cost basis, subject to TEFRA payment limita-tions and incentives. Each provi-der's reimbursement is subject to a ceiling or target amount that serves as an upper limit on operating costs. Depending upon the relation-ship of the hospital's actual costs to its target amount, these hospitals may receive relief or bonus pay-ments as well as additional bonus payments for continuous improve-ment (i.e., facilities whose costs have been consistently less than their limits may receive additional money). Newly established hospitals receive special treatment. Providers that can demonstrate that there has been a significant change	An update factor for reimburse-ment of operating costs is established by statute. Starting in FY2006, the IPPS operating MB increase is used to update the target amounts. The amount of increase received by any specific hospital will depend upon the relationship of the hospital's costs to its target amount. There is no specific update for capital costs.	The update for **FY2009** was 3.6%. The update for **FY2010** is 2.1%.

Table 3. (Continued)

Provider/service	General payment policy	General update policy	Recent update
subunit of another entity); and have at least 50% of their discharges with a diagnosis of neo-plastic disease. See 42 CFR 412.23(f).	in services and/or patients may receive exceptions payments. The capital costs for these hospitals are reimbursed on a reasonable cost basis.		
Critical Access Hospitals (CAHs) are limited-service facilities that are located more than 35 miles from another hospital (15 miles in certain circums-tances) or designated by the state as a necessary provider of health care; offer 24-hour emergency care; have no more than 25 acute care inpatient beds and have a 96-hour average length of stay. Beds in	Medicare pays CAHs on the basis of the reasonable costs of the facility for inpatient and outpatient services. CAHs may elect either a cost-based hospital outpatient service payment or an all-inclusive rate which is equal to a reasonable cost payment for facility services plus 115% of the fee schedule payment for professional services. Ambulance services that are owned and operated by CAHs are reimbursed on a reasonable cost basis if these ambulance services are 35 miles from another ambulance system. MMA provided that inpatient, outpatient, and swing bed services provided by	No specific update policy.	No specific update policy.

Table 3. (Continued)

Provider/service	General payment policy	General update policy	Recent update
distinct-part skilled nursing facility, psychiatric or rehabilitation units operated by a CAH do not count toward the bed limit.	CAHs will be paid at 101% of reasonable costs for cost reporting periods beginning January 1, 2004. Starting July 1, 2009, clinical diagnostic laboratory services furnished by a CAH will be paid as outpatient hospital services at 101% of costs without regard to whether the individual is physically present in the CAH, or in a SNF or a clinic (including a rural health clinic) that is operated by a CAH at the time the specimen is collected.		

Table 4. Skilled Nursing Facility (SN F) Care

Provider/ service	General payment policy	General update policy	Recent update
Skilled Nursing Facility (SNF) care	SNFs are paid through a prospective payment system (PPS) which is composed of a daily ("per-diem") urban or rural base payment amount adjusted for case mix and area wages. The federal per diem payment is intended to cover all the services provided to the beneficiary that day, including room and board, nursing, therapy, and prescription drugs. Some costs are excluded from PPS and paid separately such as	The urban and rural federal per diem payment rates are increased annually by an update factor determined, in part, by the projected increase in the SNF market basket (MB) index. This index measures changes in the costs of goods and services purchased by SNFs. Each year, the update may include an	For **FY2009,** SNFs received the full MB increase of 3.4%.

Table 4. (Continued)

Provider/ service	General payment policy	General update policy	Recent update
	physician visits, dialysis and certain high cost prosthetics and orthotics. The case-mix adjustment to the base per diem rate adjusts payments for the treatment and care needs of Medicare beneficiaries and categorizes individuals into groups called resource utilization groups (RUGs). The RUGs system uses patient assessments to assign a beneficiary to one of 53 categories and to determine the payment for the beneficiary's care. Patient assessments are done at various times during a patient's stay and their RUG may change. The federal payment is also adjusted to account for variations in area wages, using the hospital wage index. According to the FY2010 CMS Final SNF rule, the SNF RUG-III methodology was to be replaced with a revised RUG-IV methodo-logy. For FY2010, PPACA delays the implementation of this revised RUG methodology until FY2011. Starting on October 1, 2004, MMA increased payments for AIDS patients in SNFs by 128%. Unlike other PPSs, the SNF PPS statute does not provide for an adjustment for extraordinarily costly cases (an "outlier" adjustment). DRA reduced payments to SNFs for beneficiary bad debts to 70% for non-duals (individuals who are not enrolled in both Medicare and Medicaid). Bad debt payments for dual eligibles (individuals enrolled in both Medicare and Medicaid) remain at 100%.	adjustment to account for the MB forecast error for previous years. Since FY2008, when the difference between the estimated MB update and the actual increase is greater than 0.5 percentage points, payments to SNFs are updated to account for this forecast error. When the difference is less than 0.5 percentage points, no adjustments are made. For FY2011, SNFs will receive the full MB update. Starting in FY2012, all SNF MB updates will be subject to the productivity adjustment.	For **FY2010**, SNFs receive the full MB increase of 2.2%.

Table 5. Hospice Care

Provider/ Service	General payment policy	General update policy	Recent update
Hospice care	Payments for hospice care contain three separate components that are adjusted annually. These components are the payment rates, the hospice wage index, and the cap amount. Limited cost sharing applies to outpatient drugs and respite care. **Payment rates** are based on one of four prospectively determined rates which correspond to four different levels of care (i.e., routine home care, continuous home care, inpatient respite care, and general inpatient care) for each day a beneficiary is under the care of the hospice. The **hospice wage index** is used to adjust payment rates to reflect local differences in area wage levels. This index is established using the most current hospital wage data available. Total payments to a hospice are	Each of the three components are updated annually. The prospective **payment rates** are updated by the increase in the hospice market basket (MB). Since FY2003 updates have been at the full hospital MB percentage increase. For FY2010 – FY2012, hospice providers receive the full **MB update**. For FY2013, the MB update will be reduced by 0.3% and adjusted by the productivity factor. For FY2014 – FY2019, a 0.3% reduction to the MB will be contingent upon the level of the insured population relative to the projection of the insured population for 2009. Only if the level of non-elderly insured population is 5 or fewer percentage points above the projections will the MB be reduced by 0.3%.	The **FY2009 payment rates** were updated by the MB of 3.6%. The national hospice base payment rates for care furnished during **FY2009** were as follows: routine home care— $139.97; continuous home care—$816.94 for 24 hours or $34.04 per hour; inpatient respite care—$144.79 per day; and general inpatient care—$622.66 per day. The **FY2010 payment rates** are updated by the MB of 2.1%. This update is affected by the BNAF reduction of 10% in the FY2010 Hospice Wage Index. The net effect is a 1.4% increase in payment rates. The national hospice base payment rates for care furnished during FY2010 are as follows: routine home

Table 5. (Continued)

Provider/ Service	General payment policy	General update policy	Recent update
	subject to an aggregate **cap** that is determined by multiplying the cap amount for a given year by the number of Medicare beneficiaries who receive hospice services during the year. Medicare payments to hospices that exceed this amount must be returned to the Medicare program. Not earlier than October 1, 2013, **PPACA** requires the Secretary to implement budget neutral revisions to the methodology for determining hospice payments for routine care and other services.	The **hospice wage index** is updated to reflect updates in the hospital wage index and any changes to the definition of Metropolitan Statistical Areas (MSAs). In 1997, a hospcie wage index **budget neutrality adjust-ment factor (BNAF)** was instituted to account for differences in hospice payments as a result of a change in the data source used to adjust for geographic differences in labor from the 1983 Bureau of Labor Statistics data to the **hospital wage index**. The final rule for FY2010 phases-out the BNAF over 7 years. As a result, the BNAF is reduced by 10 percent in FY2010, and 15 percent each year from FY2011 through FY2016. The hospice **cap** amount is increased or decreased annually by the same percentage as the medical care expenditure category of the CPI-U.	care— $142.91; continuous home care—$834.10 for 24 hours or $34.75 per hour; inpatient respite care—$147.83 per day; and general inpatient care—$406.94 per day. The latest hospice **cap** amount for the cap year November 2, 2008 through October 31, 2009, is an aggregated $23,014.50 per beneficiary. For the year, ending on October 31, 2008 it was an aggregated $22,386.15 per beneficiary.

Part B

Table 6. Physicians

Provider/ service	General payment policy	General update policy	Recent update
Physicians	Payments for physicians services are made on the basis of a fee schedule. The fee schedule assigns relative values to services. These relative values reflect physician work (based on time, skill, and intensity involved), practice expenses (including the cost of nurses and other staff), and malpractice expenses. The relative values are adjusted for geographic variations in the costs of practicing medicine. These geogra-phically adjusted relative values are converted into a dollar payment amount by a conversion factor. Assistants-at-surgery services (provided by physicians) are paid 16% of the	The conversion factor is updated each year by a formula specified in law. The update percentage equals the Medicare Economic Index (MEI, which measures inflation) subject to an adjustment to match spending under the cumulative sustainable growth rate (SGR) system. (The SGR is linked, in part, to changes in the gross domestic product per capita.) The adjustment sets the conversion factor so that projected spending for the year will equal allowed spending by the end of the year. Application of the SGR system led to a 5.4% reduction in the conversion factor in 2002. Additional reductions were slated to take effect in subsequent years. However, P.L. 108-7 allowed for revisions in previous	Congress has passed several bills that have overridden the reduction in the update factor that would have been required for 2010 under the SGR formula. For January 1 through May 31, the update to the conversion factor was set to 0% as a result of three separate acts. For the six months from June 1 through November 30, 2010, the update to the conversion factor is 2.2%. Unless Congress passes additional legislation, a substantial reduction in the update factor will be required on December 1, 2010. PPACA included several modifications to Medicare physician reimbursement, including bonus payments for

Table 6. (Continued)

Provider/ service	General payment policy	General update policy	Recent update
	fee schedule amount. Anesthesia services are paid under a separate fee schedule (based on base and time units) with a separate conversion factor. Medicare payments for most professional services equal 80% of the fee schedule amount; patients are liable for the remaining 20%.	estimates used for the SGR calculation, thereby permitting an update of 1.6% effective March 1, 2003. MMA provided that the update to the conversion factor for 2004 and 2005 could not be less than 1.5%. DRA froze the 2006 rate at the 2005 level, TRHCA froze the 2007 rate at the 2006 level; and MMSEA provided that the level for the first six months of 2008 is increased by 0.5%. MIPPA exten-ded this 0.5% increase through the end of 2008 and provided for a 1.1% increase in 2009. Under current law, the conversion factor update can not be more than three percentage points above nor more than seven percentage points below the MEI, however, several of the bills that have averted the SGR reductions have included language that has overridden this condition.	primary care services and for successfully reporting quality measures as well as many adjustments to the methodologies for calculating payments. (See CRS report on Medicare and PPACA for details). For many years, prior to the passage of MIPPA, beneficiary payments for outpatient mental health services equaled 50% of the fee schedule amounts. MIPPA included a mental health parity provision to be phased in over 5 years. For services provided before Jan. 1, 2010, beneficiaries pay 50% of the covered charges (after meeting their deductible); beginning Jan. 1, 2014, outpatient mental health services will be covered at the same rate (80%) as other Part B services.

Table 7. Nonphysician Practitioners

Provider/ service	General payment policy	General update policy	Recent update
(a) Physician Assistants	Separate payments are made for physician assistant (PA) services, when provided under the supervision of a physician, but only if no facility or other provider charge is paid. Payment is made to the employer (such as a physician). The PA may be in an independent contractor relationship with the employer. The recognized payment amount equals 85% of the physician fee schedule amount (or, for assistant-at-surgery services, 85% of the amount that would be paid to a physician serving as an assistant-at-surgery). Medicare payments equal 80% of this amount; patients are liable for the remaining 20%. Assignment is mandatory for PA services.	See physician fee schedule.	See physician fee schedule. In a skilled nursing facility (SNF), Medicare law allows physicians, as well as nurse practitioners and clinical nurse specialists who do not have a direct or indirect employment relationship with a SNF, but who are working in collaboration with a physician, to certify the need for post-hospital extended care services for purposes of Medicare payment. PPACA includes a provision that allows a physician assistant who does not have a direct or indirect employment relation-ship with a SNF, but who is working in collaboration with a physician, to certify the need for post-hospital extended care services for Medicare payment

Table 7. (Continued)

Provider/ service	General payment policy	General update policy	Recent update
			purposes,beginning on or after January 1, 2011.
(b) Nurse Practitioners (NPs) and Clinical Nurse Specialists (CNSs)	Separate payments are made for NP or CNS services, provided in collaboration with a physician, but only if no other facility or other provider charge is paid. The recognized payment amount equals 85% of the physician fee schedule amount (or, for assistant-at-surgery services, 85% of the amount that would be paid to a physician serving as an assistant-at-surgery). Medicare payments equal 80% of this amount; patients are liable for the remaining 20%. Assignment is mandatory.	See physician fee schedule.	See physician fee schedule.
(c) Nurse midwives	The recognized payment amount for certified nurse midwife services equals 65% of the physician fee schedule amount. Nurse midwives can be paid directly. Medicare payments equal 80% of this amount; patients are liable for the remaining 20%. Assignment is mandatory.	See physician fee schedule.	See physician fee schedule.

Table 7. (Continued)

Provider/ service	General payment policy	General update policy	Recent update
(d) Certified Registered Nurse Anesthetists (CRNAs)	CRNAs are paid under the same fee schedule used for anesthesiologists. Payments furnished by an anesthesia care team composed of an anesthesiologist and a CRNA are capped at 100% of the amount that would be paid if the anesthesiolo-gist was practicing alone. The payments are evenly split between each practitioner. CRNAs can be paid directly. Assignment is manda-tory for services provided by CRNAs. Regular Part B cost sharing applies.	See physician fee schedule.	See physician fee schedule.
(e) Clinical Psycholo-gists and Clinical Social Workers	The recognized payment amount for services provided by a clinical social worker is equal to 75% of the physician fee schedule amount. Services in connection with the treatment of mental, psychoneurotic, and personality disorders of a patient who is not a hospital inpatient are subject to the mental health services limitation. In these cases Medicare pays 50% of incurred expenses and the patient is liable for the remaining 50%. Otherwise, regular Part	See physician fee schedule.	See physician fee schedule.

Table 7. (Continued)

Provider/ service	General payment policy	General update policy	Recent update
	B cost sharing applies. Assignment is mandatory for services provided by clinical psychologists and clinical social workers.		
(f) Outpatient physical or occupational therapy services	Payments are made under the physician fee schedule. Medicare coverage for outpatient therapy services, including physical therapy, speech-language pathology services, and occupational therapy have limits or "caps." To accommodate patients with therapy needs that exceed the cap, Congress created an exceptions process that allows for specific diagnoses and procedures to receive Medicare coverage even after a beneficiary has met the therapy cap for the year. In 1999, an annual $1,500 per beneficiary limit applied to all outpatient physical therapy services (including speech-language pathology services), except for those furnished by a hospital outpatient department. A separate $1,500 limit applied to all outpatient occupational	Updates in fee schedule payments are dependent on the update applicable under the physician fee schedule. The $1,500 limits were to be increased by the increase in the MEI beginning in 2002; however, application of the limits was suspended until September 1, 2003. At that time the limits were $1,590. MMA suspended the application of the limits beginning December 8, 2003-December 31, 2005. The limits were restored January 1, 2006. DRA required the Secretary to establish an exceptions process for 2006 for certain medically	See physician fee schedule. The CY2009 limits or "caps" were $1,840. The CY2010 limits are $1,860. However, the Temporary Extension Act of 2010, H.R. 4691 extended the exceptions process through March 31, 2010 and PPACA extended the exceptions process for therapy caps through December 31, 2010.

Table 7. (Continued)

Provider/ service	General payment policy	General update policy	Recent update
	therapy services except for those furnished by hospital outpatient departments. Therapy services furnished as incident to physicians professional services were included in these limits. The $1,500 limits were to apply each year. However, no limits applied from 2000-2005, except for a brief period in 2003. The limits were restored in 2006; however, an exceptions process has applied in each year since the limits were reintroduced in 2006. Regular Part B cost sharing applies. Assignment is optional for services provided by therapists in independent practice; balance billing limits apply for non-assigned claims. Assignment is mandatory for other therapy services.	necessary services. TRHCA extended the exceptions process through 2007; MMSEA extended the process an additional six months. MIPPA extended the exceptions process through December 31, 2009. The limits were $1,780, the 2008 limits were $1,810, and the 2009 limits were $1,840.2006 limits were $1,740; the 2007	

Table 8. Clinical Diagnostic Laboratory Services

Provider/ service	General payment policy	General update policy	Recent update
Clinical diagnostic laboratory services	Clinical lab services are paid on the basis of area-wide fee schedules. The fee schedule amounts are periodically updated. There is a ceiling on payment amounts equal to 74% of the median of all fee schedules for the test. Assignment is mandatory. No cost sharing is imposed.	Generally, the Secretary of HHS is required to adjust the payment amounts annually by the percentage change in the CPI, together with such other adjustments as the Secretary deems appropriate. Updates were eliminated for 1998 through 2002. MMA eliminated updates for 2004-2008. The annual clinical laboratory test fee schedule update adjustment for 2009-2013 will be the percentage increase or decrease in the CPI for all urban consumers minus 0.5 percentage points. MIPPA repealed the Medicare Competitive Bidding Demonstration Project for Clinical Laboratory Services. MIPAA clarified the payment for clinical laboratory services in CAHs. Beginning July 1, 2009, clinical diagnostic laboratory services furnished by a CAH will be reimbursed as outpatient hospital services at 101% of costs without regard to whether the individual who receives the service is physically present in the CAH, or in a skilled nursing home or a clinic (including a rural health clinic) that is operated by a CAH at the time the specimen is collected.	The fee schedules were updated by 1.1% in 2003. Per MMA, no update was made for 2004, 2005, 2006, 2007, or 2008. In 2009, the update was 4.5%. For 2010, the update is - 1.9%. PPACA modified provider updates based on the MB or CPI minus full productivity estimates for all Parts A and B providers and suppliers who are subject to a MB or CPI update. (See above for details.) For the clinical laboratory test fee schedule, the modification will replace the scheduled 0.5% payment reduction for CY2011 through CY2013 with a fullproductivity adjustment for CY2011 and subsequent years. A 1.75 percentage point reduction to the update in CY2011 through CY2015 will be established; this reduction may result in a negative update. The productivity adjustment factor will be applied to the CPI-U starting in CY2011, but in the application of the adjustment will not be able to reduce the increase to less than zero. PPACA authorized a two-year demon-stration project, beginning on July 1, 2011, that will make separate payments to laboratories for complex diagnostic laboratory tests provided to Medicare beneficiaries and provided a one year extension (ending July 1, 2011) for clinical diagnostic laboratory service for qualifying rural hospitals with under 50 beds to be paid on the basis of reasonable cost.

Table 9. Preventive Services

Provider/ service	General payment policy	General update policy	Recent update
Pap smears; pelvic exams	Medicare covers screening pap smears and screening pelvic exams once every two years; annual coverage is authorized for women at high risk. Payment is based on the clinical diagnostic laboratory fee schedule. Assignment is mandatory. No cost sharing is imposed.	See clinical laboratory fee schedule. A national Minimum payment amount applies for pap smears.	See clinical laboratory fee schedule. Minimum payment for pap smears in 2010 is $15.13 (down 1.9%, or $0.29, from 2009).
Screening mammograms	Coverage is authorized for an annual screening mammogram. Payment is made under the physician fee schedule. The deductible is waived; regular Part B coinsurance applies. Assignment is optional. Balance billing limits apply on non-assigned claims.	See physician fee schedule.	See physician fee schedule.
Colorectal screening	Coverage is provided for the following procedures for the early detection of colon cancer: (1) screening fecal occult blood tests (for persons over 50, no more than annually); (2) screening flexible sigmoidoscopy (for persons over 50, no more than once every four years and 10 years after a screening colonoscopy for those not at high risk for colon cancer); (3) screening flexible colonoscopy for high-risk individuals (limited to one every two years) and for those not at high risk, every 10 years or four years after a screening sigmoidoscopy; and (4) barium enemas (as an alternative to either a	See physician fee schedule and laboratory fee schedule.	See physician fee schedule and laboratory fee schedule.

Table 9. (Continued)

Provider/ service	General payment policy	General update policy	Recent update
	screening flexible sigmoidoscopy or screening colonoscopy in accordance with the same screening parameters established for those tests). Payments are based on rates paid for the same procedure when done for a diagnostic purpose. Fecal occult blood tests are paid under the laboratory fee schedule; other tests are paid under physician fee schedule. If a sigmoidoscopy or colonoscopy results in a biopsy or removal of a lesion, it would be classified and paid as the procedure with such biopsy or removal, rather than as a diagnostic test. Assignment is mandatory for fecal occult blood tests and no cost sharing applies. Assignment is optional for sigmoidoscopies and colonoscopies. DRA specified that the Part B deductible does not apply for screenings, effective January 1, 2007. Balance billing limits apply on non-assigned claims.		
Prostate cancer screening	Medicare covers an annual prostate cancer screening test. Payment is made under the physician fee schedule.	See physician fee schedule.	See physician fee schedule.
Glaucoma screening	Medicare covers an annual glaucoma screening for persons with diabetes, persons with a family history of glaucoma, African-Americans age 50 and over, and	See physician fee schedule.	See physician fee schedule.

Table 9. (Continued)

Provider/ service	General payment policy	General update policy	Recent update
	Hispanic Americans age 65 and over. Payment is made under the physician fee schedule.		
Diabetes outpatient self-management training	Medicare covers services furnished by a certified provider. Payment is made under the physician fee schedule.	See physician fee schedule.	See physician fee schedule.
Medical nutrition therapy services	Coverage is authorized for certain individuals with diabetes or renal disease. Payment equals 85% of the amount established under the physician fee schedule for the service if it had been furnished by a physician.	See physician fee schedule.	See physician fee schedule.
Bone mass measurements	Bone mass measurements are covered for certain high-risk individuals. Payments are made under the physician fee schedule. In general, services are covered if they are provided no more frequently than once every two years.	See physician fee schedule.	See physician fee schedule.
Ultrasound screenings for abdominal aortic aneurysms	Ultrasound screenings for abdominal aortic aneurysms are covered for individuals who: (1) receive a referral for such screening during the initial preventive services exam; (2) have not had such a screening paid for by Medicare; and (3) have a family history of abdominal aortic aneurysm or manifest certain risk factors.	See physician fee schedule.	See physician fee schedule.

Table 10. Telehealth

Provider/Service	General payment policy	General update policy	Recent update
Telehealth services	Medicare pays for services furnished via a telecommunications system by a physician or practitioner, notwithstanding the fact that the individual providing the service is not at the same location as the beneficiary. Payment is equal to the amount that would be paid under the physician fee schedule if the service had been furnished without a telecommunications system. A facility fee is paid to the originating site (the site where the beneficiary is when the service is provided).	Current law established the pay-ment amount for the Medicare telehealth originating site facility fee for telehealth services provided from October 1, 2001 through December 31, 2002 at $20. The facility fee for telehealth services provided on or after January 1 of each subsequent calendar year is the amount for the previous year increased as of the first day of the subsequent year by the percentage increase in the Medicare Economic Index (MEI). MIPPA added certain entities as originating sites eligible for for payment of telehealth services. Eligible distant site physicians and practitioners who provide services to beneficiaries located at the expanded list of sites may now be paid for qualifying telehealth services. This expanded list includes hospital-based or critical access hospital-based renal dialysis centers (including satellites); skilled nursing facilities (SNFs); and/or community mental health centers (CMHCs.)	See physician fee schedule. The MEI increase for CY2010 is 1.2% and the telehealth originating site facility fee for CY2010 is 80% of the lesser of the actual charge or $24.00 (compared to $23.72 in CY2009).

Table 11. Durable Medical Equipment (DME)

Provider/ service	General payment policy	General update policy	Recent update
Durable Medical Equipment (DME)	Except in designated DMEPOS Competitive Bidding Areas, DME is paid on the basis of a fee schedule. Items are classified into five groups for determining the fee schedules and making payments: (1) inexpensive or other routinely purchased equipment (defined as items costing less than $150 or which are purchased at least 75% of the times); (2) items requiring frequent and substantial servicing; (3) customized items; (4) oxygen and oxygen equipment; and (5) other items referred to as capped rental items. In general, fee schedule rates are established locally and are subject to national limits. The national limits have floors and ceilings. The floor is equal to 85% of the weighted average of all local payment amounts and the ceiling is equal to 100% of the weighted average of all local payment amounts. Assignment is optional. Balance billing limits do not apply on non-assigned claims.	In general, fee schedule amounts are updated annually by the CPI-U. Updates were eliminated for 1998-2000; payments were increased by the CPI-U for 2001; and payments were frozen for 2002. MMA eliminated the updates for 2004-2008. To pay for the delay in the competitive acquisition program, MIPPA reduced the fee schedule update for 2009 by 9.5% for all items, services and accessories included in round 1 of the competitive bidding program. For 2010 the fee schedule update will be the increase in the CPI-U.. Starting in 2011 PPACA requires the fee schedule	The update for **CY2003** was 1.1%. As required by MMA, there were no updates for **CY2004, CY2005, CY2006, CY2007,** and **CY2008.** In **CY2009**, the following 10 items were subject to a 9.5% reduction: oxygen supplies and equipment; standard power wheelchairs, scooters and related accessories; complex rehabilitative power wheelchairs and related accessories; mail-order diabetic supplies; enteral nutrients, equipment, and supplies; continuous positive airway pressure (CPAP) devices and Respiratory Assist Devices (RADs) and related supplies; hospital beds and related accessories; negative pressure wound therapy pumps and related supplies and accessories; walkers

Table 11. (Continued)

Provider/ service	General payment policy	General update policy	Recent update
	Regular Part B cost sharing applies.MMA required the Secretary to begin a program of competitive acquisition for DME, prosthetics and orthotics in which payments for these items would be based on the bids of winning suppliers. Competitive acquisition was to begin in 10 metropolitan statistical areas (MSAs) in 2007, expanding to 80 MSAs in 2008, and additional areas in 2009. The first round of bids were submitted on September 25, 2007, and the program began on July 1, 2008. However, MIPPA stopped the program, terminated all contracts with suppliers and required the Secretary to rebid the first round in 2009. Expansion of the program was delayed by two years until 2011. FPACA expan-ded the number of areas in round two to 91 and requires the Secre-tary to expand the program or apply competitive rates to remain-ing areas by 2016.	update for DME to be subject to a productivity adjustment, which may result in a negative update.	and related accessories; and support surfaces, including group 2 mattresses and overlays. In **CY2009,** all items not subject to the 9.5% reduction received a 5.0% update. For the **CY2010** update, the CPI-U for the applicable period is -1.4%, however Medicare set the update at 0.0%.

Table 12. Prosthetics and Orthotics

Provider/service	General payment policy	General update policy	Recent update
Prosthetics and orthotics	Except in designated DMEPOS competitive bidding areas as described above, prosthetics and orthotics are paid on the basis of a fee schedule. These rates are established regionally and are subject to national limits which have floors and ceilings. The floor is equal to 90% of the weighted average of all regional payment amounts and the ceiling is equal to 120% of the weighted average of all regional payment amounts. Assignment is optional; balance billing limits do not apply on non-assigned claims. Regular Part B cost sharing applies.	Fee schedule amounts are updated annually by the CPI-U. MMA eliminated the updates for 2004-2006. Starting in 2011 PPACA requires the fee schedule update for prosthetics and orthotics to be subject to a productivity adjustment, which may result in negative update.	The update for **CY2003** was 1.1%. As required by MMA, there were no updates for **CY2004, CY2005** and **CY2006.** The update for **CY2007** was 4.3%. The update for CY2008 was 2.7%. The update for **CY2009** was 5.0%. For the **CY2010** update, the CPI-U for the applicable period is -1.4%, however Medicare set the update at 0.0%.

Table 13. Surgical Dressings

Provider/service	General payment policy	General update policy	Recent update
Surgical Dressings	Surgical dressings are paid on the basis of a fee schedule. Payment levels are computed using the same methodology as the durable medical equipment fee schedule (see above). Assignment is optional; balance billing limits do not apply to non-assigned claims. Regular Part B cost sharing applies.	See durable medical equipment fee schedule. Starting in 2011 PPACA requires the fee schedule update for medical supplies to be subject to a productivity adjustment, which may result in negative update.	The update for CY2003 was 1.1%. There was no update for CY2004, CY2005, CY2006, CY2007, and CY2008. The update for CY2009 was 5.0%. For the CY2010 update, the CPI-U for the applicable period is -1.4%, however Medicare set the update at 0.0%.

Table 14. Parenteral and Enteral Nutrition (PEN)

Provider/service	General payment policy	General update policy	Recent update
Parenteral and Enteral Nutrition (PEN)	Except in designated DMEPOS competitive bidding areas as described above, parenteral and enteral nutrients, equipment, and supplies are paid on the basis of the PEN fee schedule. Prior to 2002, PEN was paid on a reasonable charge basis (see below under Miscellane-ous Items and Services). The fee schedule amounts are based on payment amounts made on a national basis to PEN suppliers under the reasonable charge system. Assignment is optional; balance billing limits do not apply on non-assigned claims. Regular Part B cost sharing applies.	Fee schedule amounts are updated annually by the CPI-U. MIPPA reduced the fee schedule update for 2009 by 9.5% for all items, services and accessories included in round 1 of the competitive bidding program. Enteral nutrition was included in the first round of competitive bidding, and is thus subject to the 9.5% fee schedule reduction in CY2009. Parenteral nutrition was not included in round 1. Starting in 2011 PPACA requires the fee schedule update for parenteral and enteral nutrition to be subject to a productivity adjustment, which may result in a negative update.	In **CY2009** Enteral nutrients, equipment and supplies were subject to the 9.5% reduction while parenteral nutrients received a 5.0% update. For the **CY2010** update, the CPI-U for the applicable period is -1.4%, however Medicare set the update at 0.0%.

Table 15. Miscellaneous Items and Services

Provider/service	General payment policy	General update policy	Recent update
Miscellaneous services	Miscellaneous items and services here refers to those services still paid on a reasonable charge basis. Included are such items as splints, casts, home dialysis supplies and equipment, therapeutic shoes, certain intraocular lenses, and transfusion medicine. These charges may not exceed any of the following fee screens: (1) the supplier's customary charge for the item, (2) the prevailing charge for the item in the locality, (3) the charges made to the carrier's policyholders or subscribers for comparable items, (4) the inflation-indexed charge. Assignment is optional; balance billing limits do not apply on non-assigned claims. Regular Part B cost sharing applies.	Payments for reasonable charge items are calculated annually. Carriers determine a supplier's customary charge level. Prevailing charges may not be higher than 75% of the customary charges made for similar items and services in the locality during the 12-month period of July 1-June 30 of the previous calendar year. The inflation-indexed charge is updated by the CPI-U.	The update to the inflation-indexed charge for **CY2007** was 4.3%. The update to the inflation-indexed charge for **CY2008** was 2.7%. The **CY2009** update was 5.0%. For the CY2010 update, the CPI-U for the applicable period is - 1.4%, however Medicare set the update at 0.0%.

Table 16. Ambulatory Surgical Centers (ASCs)

Provider/service	General Payment policy	General update policy	Recent update
Ambulatory Surgical Centers (ASCs)	Starting January 1, 2008, Medicare will pay for surgery-related facility services provided in an ASC using a payment system based on the hospital outpatient prospective payment system (OPPS). The new payment system will be implemen-ted over a four-year transition period. The ASC payment system uses the same payment groups (APCs) as the OPPS. Many of the ASC relative weights procedures will be the same as in OPPS. Certain services will be eligible for separate payments. The relative weights will be multiplied by a conversion factor (average payment amount) to get a payment for a specific procedure. The ASC conversion factor is based on a percentage of the OPPS conversion factor set to ensure budget neutrality between the old ASC payment system and the new one. CMS uses different methods to set payments for new office-based procedures, separately payable radiology services, separately payable drugs and device intensive services.	MMA eliminated the payment update for FY2005 under the prior payment system, changed the update cycle to a calendar year from a fiscal year, and eliminated the updates for calendar years 2006-2009. MMA also established that a revised pay-ment system for surgical services furnished in an ASC will be imple-mented on or after January 1, 2006, and not later than January 1, 2008. Total payments under the new system should be equal to the total projected payments under the old system. As established by the TRHCA, starting in CY2009, the annual increase for ASCs that do not submit required quality data may be the required update minus 2 percentage points. The reduction for not submitting quality data would apply for the applicable year only, and not for subsequent years. Beginning in CY2010, the ASC conversion factor will be updated annually using the consumer price index for all urban consumers (CPI-U). The ASC update will include a productivity adjustment starting January 1, 2011.	In **CY2009**, the ASC conversion factor was established at $41.393, after budget neutrality adjustments. The **CY2010** update of 1.2% is subject to a wage index budget neutrality adjustment of 0.9996. The CY2010 ASC conversion factor is $41.873.

Table 17. Hospital Outpatient Services

Provider/service	General payment policy	General update policy	Recent update
Hospital Outpatient Departments (HOPDs)	Under HOPD-PPS, which was implemented in August 2000, the unit of payment is the individual service or procedure as assigned to one of about 570 ambulatory payment classifications (APCs). To the extent possible, integral services and items are bundled within each APC, specified new technologies are assigned to new technology APCs until clinical and cost data is available to permit assignment into a clinical APC. Medicare's payment for HOPD services is calculated by multiplying the relative weight associated with an APC by a conversion factor. For most APCs, 60% of the conversion factor is geographi-cally adjusted by the IPPS wage index. Except for new technology APCs, each APC has a relative weight that is based on the median cost of services in that APC. Certain APCs with significant fluctuations in their relative weights will have the calculated change dampened. The HOPD-PPS also includes budget-neutral pass-through payments for new technology and budget-neutral outlier payments. Cancer and children's hospitals have a permanent hold	The conversion factor is updated on a calendar year schedule. These annual updates are based on the hospital IPPS MB. As established by TRHCA, starting in CY2009, the update for hospitals that do not submit required quality data will be the MB minus 2 percentage points. The reduction for not submitting quality data would apply for the applicable year, and would not be taken into account in subsequent years. PPACA established a schedule of annual reductions in the update for starting CY2010 through CY2019. The CY2010 update reduction is 0.25 percentage points.	For **CY2009**, the update was 3.6%. Hospitals that fail to submit the required quality data l received an update of 1.6%. This increase was adjusted by budget-neutrality factors associated with wage index changes and pass through expenses. The final CY2009 conversion factor for hospitals that did submit the required quality data was \$66.059 and was \$64.784 for those that did not submit the required data. For **CY2010**, the MB update is 2.1% which, as directed by PPACA, is re-duced by 0.25 percentage points to

Table 17. (Continued)

Provider/service	General payment policy	General update policy	Recent update
	harmless protection from the HOPD-PPS. HOPDs in rural hospitals with 100 or fewer beds (that are not SCHs) will receive at least 85% of the payment it would have received under the prior payment system during CY2010. Starting for services on January 1, 2006, rural SCHs will receive a 7.1% payment increase. All SCHs receive 85% of the payment difference for covered HOPD services furnished during CY2010. Over time, under Medicare's prior payment system, beneficiaries' share of total outpatient payments grew to 50%. HOPD-PPS slowly reduces the beneficiary's copayment for these services. Copayments will be frozen at 20% of the national median charge for the service in 1996, updated to 1999. Over time, as PPS amounts rise, the frozen Beneficiary copayments will decline as a share of the total payment until the beneficiary share is 20% of the Medicare fee schedule amount. A beneficiary copayment amount for a procedure is limited to the inpatient deductible amount established for that year. Balance billing is prohibited.	The update will include a productivity adjustment starting January 1, 2012. The PPACA update reductions may result in a negative update for that year.	result in an increase in 1.85%. Hospitals that did not submit required quality data receive a negative 0.15% update. This increase was adjusted by the required budget neutrality factors for wage index changes and pass-through expenses. The CY2010 conversion factor is $67.241 for hospitals that submit required quality data and $65.921 for hospitals that did not submit this data. (The prior year's update penalty for not submitting quality data is not taken into account in the next year.)

Table 18. Rural Health Clinics and Federally Qualified Health Center (FQHCs) Services

Provider/service	General payment policy	General update policy	Recent update
Rural Health Clinics (RHCs) and Federally Qualified Health Center (FQHCs) services	RHCs and FQHCs are paid on the basis of an all-inclusive rate for each beneficiary visit for covered services. An interim payment is made to the RHC or FQHC based on estimates of allowable costs and number of visits; a reconcilia-tion is made at the end of the year based on actual costs and visits. Per-visit payment limits are established for all RHCs (other than those in hospitals with fewer than 50 beds) and FHQCs. Assignment is mandatory; no deductible applies for FHQC services.	Payment limits are updated on January 1 of each year by the Medicare economic index (MEI) which measures inflation for certain medical services.	For **CY2009**, the RHC upper payment limit was $76.84, the urban FQHC limit was $119.29, and the rural FQHC limit was $102.58. For **CY2010,** the RHC upper payment limit is $77.76, the urban FQHC limit is $125.72, and the rural FQHC limit is $108.81.

Table 19. Comprehensive Outpatient Rehabilitation Facility (CORF)

Provider/service	General payment policy	General update policy	Recent update
Comprehensive Outpatient Rehabilitation Facility (CORF)	CORFs provide (by or under the supervision of physicians) outpatient diagnostic, therapeutic and restorative services. Payments for services are made on the basis of the physician fee schedule. Therapy services are subject to the therapy limits (described above for physical and occupational therapy providers).	See physician fee schedule and outpatient physical and occupational therapy services.	See physician fee schedule and outpatient physical and occupational therapy services.

Table 20. Part B Drugs and Biologicals Covered Incident to a Physician's Visit

Provider/service	General payment policy	General update policy	Recent update
Drugs and biologics including vaccines. Medicare covers certain outpatient drugs and biologicals under the Part B program that are authorized by statute, including those: (1) that are covered if they are usually not self-administered and are provided incident to a physician's services; (2) those that are necessary for the effective use of covered DME; (3) certain self-administered oral cancer and antinausea drugs (those	Drug products, except for pneumococcal, influenza, and hepatitis B vaccines, those associated with certain renal dialysis services, blood products and clotting factors and radiopharmaceuticals, are paid using the average sales price (ASP) methodology. The ASP for all drug products included within the same billing and payment code, usually the Healthcare Common Procedure Coding System (HCPCS) Code, is the volume-weighted average of the manufacturer's average sales prices reported to CMS across all the National Drug Codes (NDCs) assigned to the code. Medicare's payment under the ASP methodology equals 106% of the applicable price for a multiple source drug or single source drug subject to beneficiary deductible	The ASP is updated quarterly by the Secretary. Payments under the ASP method may be lowered by the Secretary if the ASP exceeds the widely available market price or average manufacturer price by a specified percentage (5% in 2006 to present, as determined by the Secretary). In such cases, the payment would equal the lesser of the widely available market price or 103% of the average manufacturer price. Several OIG reports found that the percentage was exceeded for some drugs and the Secretary has chosen not to exercise the option of lowering the payment rate for these drugs. CAP payments are updated on an annual basis based on the approved CAP vendor's reasonable net acquisition costs	According to the Centers for Medicare and Medicaid Services, the third quarter 2010 ASP payment amounts remain stable compared to the previous quarter. For most of the higher volume drugs (31 out of the top 50), the prices changed 2% or less. Overall, the prices for 13 of the top 50 drugs decrea-sed, 2 remained the same, and 35 increased. On September 10, 2008, the Centers for Medicare & Medicaid Services announced the postpone-ment of CAP program due to their inability to establish contracts with any qualified bidders.

Table 20. (Continued)

Provider/service	General payment policy	General update policy	Recent update
with injectable equivalents); (4) erythropoietin stimulating agents (ESAs) used to treat anemia; (5) immunosuppressive drugs after covered Medicare organ transplants; (6) hemophilia clotting factors; and (7) vaccines for influenza, pneumonia, and hepatitis B.	and coinsurance amounts. This is intended to cover both the acquisition cost of the drug and any adminis-trative overhead resulting from procurement, storage, and administration of the drug. Regular Part B cost sharing applies, except for pneumo-coccal and influenza virus vaccines. The MMA established a competitive acquisition program (CAP) for Medicare Part B drugs and biologicals not paid on a cost or pros-pective payment system basis. Payment amounts for drugs furnished during the first year of an approved CAP vendor's contract are set through a competitive process using bidders' prices, which use the ASP payment amounts as a ceiling. To date, BioScrip was the only bidder to sign a contract under the CAP program, however the contract expired.	based, in part, on information disclosed to CMS and limited by the weighted payment amount established under section 1847A of the Social Security Act. Adjustment to the payment amounts may be made more often than annually, but no more often than quarterly, in any of the following cases: (1) Introduction of new drugs, (2) Expiration of a drug patent or availability of a generic drug, (3) Material shortage that results in a significant price increase for the drug, or (4) Withdrawal of a drug from the market.	

Table 21. Blood

Provider/service	General payment policy	General update policy	Recent update
Blood	Medicare pays the reasonable cost for pints of blood, starting with the fourth pint, and blood components that are provided to a hospital outpatient as part of other services. (Blood that is received in an IPPS hospital is bundled into the DRG payment.) For IPPS-excluded hospitals, Medicare pays allowable costs for blood. Beneficiary pays for first three pints of blood (for Parts A and B combined) in a year, after which regular Part B cost sharing applies.	There is no specific update for the reimbursement of Part B blood costs. The outpatient facility is paid 100% of its reasonable costs as reported on its cost-reports. See the section on IPPS hospitals for updates for blood included as part of these hospitals.	No specific update.

Table 22. Partial Hospitalization Services Connected to Treatment of Mental Illnes

Provider/ service	General payment policy	General update policy	Recent update
Partial hospitalization services connected to treatment of mental illness	Medicare provides Part B hospital outpatient care payments for "partial hospitalization" mental health care. The services are covered only if the individual would otherwise require inpatient psychiatric care. Services must be provided under a structured program which is hospital-based or hospital-affiliated and must be a distinct and organized intensive ambulatory treatment service offering less than 24-hour daily care. The program may also be covered when provided in a community mental health center. Payment for professional services is made under the physician fee schedule. Other services are paid under the hospital outpatient prospective payment system. Regular Part B cost sharing applies; balance billing is prohibited.	See physician fee schedule and hospital outpatient services.	See physician fee schedule and hospital outpatient services.

Table 23. Ambulance Services

Provider/ service	General payment policy	General update policy	Recent update
Ambulance services	Ambulance services are paid on the basis of a national fee schedule, which is being phased-in. The fee schedule establishes seven categories of ground ambulance services and two categories of air ambulance services. The ground ambulance categories are: basic life support (BLS), both emergency and nonemergency; advanced life support Level 1 (ALS1), both emergency and nonemergency; advanced life support Level 2 (ALS2); specialty care transport (SCT); and paramedic ALS intercept (PI). The air ambulance categories are: fixed wing air ambulance (FW) and rotary wing air ambulance (RW). The national fee schedule is fully phased-in for air ambulance services. For ground ambulance services, payments through 2009 are equal to the greater of the national fee schedule or a blend of the national and regional fee schedule amounts. The portion of the blend based on national rates is 80% for 2007-2009. In 2010 and subsequently, the payments in all areas will be based on the national fee schedule amount. The payment for a service equals a base rate for the level of service plus payment for mileage. Geographic adjustments are made to a portion of the base rate. For ambulance services provided between July 1, 2008 and December 31, 2010, the fee schedule amounts are increased by 2% for services originating in urban areas and by 3% for services originating in rural areas. For the period July 1, 2004 to December 31, 2010, mileage payments are increased by 22.6% for ground ambulance services originating in rural, low population density areas. There is a 25% bonus on the mileage rate for trips of 51 miles and more from July 2004-December 2008. MIPPA and extended by PPACA specifies that any area designated as rural for the purposes of making payments for air ambulance services on December 31, 2006, will be treated as rural for the purpose of making air ambulance payments during the period July 1, 2008-December 31, 2010. Regular Part B cost sharing applies. Assignment is mandatory.	The fee schedule amounts are updated each year by the CPI-U for the 12 month period ending in June. The update is referred to as the ambulance inflation factor (AIF).	The CPI-U for the applicable period was -1.4%; Medicare set that the AIF for 2010 at 0.0%. The AIF for 2009 was 5.0%.

Table 24. Home Health

Provider /service	General payment policy	General update policy	Recent update
Home health services	Home health agencies (HHAs) are paid under a prospective payment system that began in FY2001. Payment is based on 60-day episodes of care for beneficiaries, subject to several adjustments, with unlimited episodes of care in a year. The payment covers skilled nursing, therapy, medical social services, aide visits, medical supplies, and others. Durable medical equipment is not included in the home health (HH) PPS. The base pay-ment amount is adjusted for: (1) diff-erences in area wages using the hospital wage index; (2) differences in the care needs of patients (case mix) using "home health resource groups" (HHRGs); (3) outlier visits (for the extraordinarily costly patients); (4) a significant change in a beneficiary's condition (SCIC); (5) a partial episode for when a beneficiary transfers from one HHA to another during a 60-day episode; (6) budget neutrality; and (7) a low utilization payment adjustment (LUPA) for beneficiaries who receive four or fewer visits. There is no difference between urban and rural base	The base payment amount, or national standardized 60-day episode rate, is increased annually by an up-date factor that is determined, in part, by the projected increase in the HH market basket (MB) index. This index measures changes in the costs of goods and services purchased by HHAs. In CY2010, HHAs receive the full MB update. As specified in PPACA, the MB updates will be reduced by 1.0% for all HHAs in CY2011 through CY2013. For CY2014, HHAs will receive the full MB. Starting in CY2015, the MB update will be subject to the productivity factor adjustment. DRA specified that HHAs that submit health care quality data, as specified by the Secretary, receive a full MB increase; while HHAs that do not submit such data receive an update equivalent to the MB minus 2 percent-age points. This requirement was applicable for CY2007 and each subsequent year. In CY2008, refinements to the Medicare HH PPS included a reduction in the national	For CY2009, the HH MB update was 2.9% for HHAs that submitted the required quality data and 0.9% for those that do not. The CY2009 base payment amounts for 60-day episode were also adjusted downward by 2.75% as a result of case mix refinements. **For CY2010**, the HH MB update is 2.0% for HHAs that submit the required quality data and 0% for HHAs that do not. The CY2010 base payment amounts for 60-day episodes were also adjusted

Table 24. (Continued)

Provider /service	General payment policy	General update policy	Recent update
	payment amounts. The HHRG applicable to a beneficiary is determined following an assessment of the patient's condition and care needs using the Outcome and Assessment Information Set (OASIS). After the assessment, a beneficiary is categorized in one of 80 HHRGs that reflect the beneficiary's clinical severity, functional status, and service requirements. Starting in CY2010, outlier payments are capped at 10% of total payments per HHA, and no more than 2.5% of total aggregate PPS payments for all Medicare HH payments. HHAs are paid 60% of the case-mix and wage-adjusted payment after submitting a request for anticipated payment (RAP). The RAP may be submitted at the beginning of a beneficiary's care once the HHA has received verbal orders from the beneficiary's physician and the assessment is completed. The remaining payment is made when the beneficiary's care is completed or the 60-day episode ends.	standardized 60-day episode payment rate for 4 years (ending in FY2011) to account for changes in case mix that are not related to home health patients' actual clinical conditions; among other things. This resulted in a payment downward for a 60-day episode of care of 2.75% for CY2008 through CY2010, and 2.71% for CY2011. According to PPACA, starting in CY2014, the Secretary is required to rebase HH payments by a percentage considered appropriate by the Secretary to, among other things, reflect the number, mix and level of intensity of HH services in an episode, and the average cost of providing care. Any adjustments that result must be made before the annual payment updates are applied for that year (see next column regarding MB updates). A four-year phase-in, ending in 2017, will be implemented, in equal increments, each increment may not exceed 3.5% of the HH PPS base payment amount as of March 23, 2010. PPACA also requires the Secretary to reduce the standard HHRG amounts such that the aggregate reduction in payments will equal 5% of total PPS payments for a period.	downward by 2.75% as a result of case mix refinements. For visits ending on or after **April 1, 2010**, and before **January 1, 2016,** HHAs serving rural areas will receive a 3% add-on payment.

Table 25. End-Stage Renal Disease Dialysis Services

Provider/ service	General payment policy	General update policy	Recent update
End-stage renal disease (ESRD)	ESRD is a condition of permanent kidney failure, that must be treated either with a kidney transplant or by dialysis. Because of the scarcity of available kidneys for transplant, dialysis is the treatment option for most ESRD beneficiaries. Dialysis treatment removed excess fluid and toxins from the patient's blood. Dialysis services involve several procedures and prescription drugs necessary to fully treat ESRD. Dialysis services are offered in three outpatient settings: hospital-based facilities, independent facilities, and the patient's home. There are two payment methods. Under Method I, facilities are paid a prospectively set amount, known as the composite rate, for each dialysis session, regardless of whether services are provided at the facility or in the patient's home. The composite rate is derived from audited cost data and	MMA provided for an update to the composite rate beginning January 1, 2005. Since April 1, 2005 the composite rate has been case-mixed adjusted, budget neutrally. The Secretary was required to update the basic wage-adjusted case-mix payment amounts annually beginning with 2006, but only for that portion of the case- mix adjusted system that is represented by the add-on adjustment and not for the portion represented by the composite rate. MIPPA changed the payment increases for the composite rate in 2009 and 2010. As required by MIPPA, estimated Medicare total dialysis payments for 2011 will equal 98% of payments that would have been made if the bundled payment system had not been	For **CY2009,** the composite rate was increased by 1% to $133.81 for both hospital-based facilities and independent facilities. The drug add-on adjustment to the composite rate payment was $20.33 per treatment. The wage index adjustment for 2009 reflected the latest available wage date, including a revised budget neutrality adjustment of 1.056672. The ESRD wage index floor was reduced from .75 to .70. Beginning in 2009, wage adjustments will be based on 100% of the Core-Based Statistical Area geographic adjustments. The composite rate for dialysis services furnished in **CY2010** increased by 1% over the

Table 25. (Continued)

Provider/ service	General payment policy	General update policy	Recent update
	adjusted for the national proportion of patients dialyzing at home versus in a facility, and for area wage differences. Beneficiaries electing home dialysis may choose not to be associated with a facility and may make independent arrangements with a supplier for equipment, supplies,and support services. Payment to these suppliers, known as Method II, is made on the basis of reasonable charges, limited to 100% of the median hospital composite rate, except for patients on continuous cycling peritoneal dialysis, when the limit is 130% of the median hospital composite rate. Assignment is mandatory; regular Part B cost sharing applies. Kidney transplan-tation services, to the extent they are inpatient hospital services, are subject to the PPS. However, kidney acquisition costs are paid on a reasonable cost basis. MMA required the Secretary to establish a basic case-mix adjusted	implemented. Per MIPPA, beginning in 2012, the Secretary will annually increase the bundled payment amounts by an ESRD market basket increase factor appropriate for a bundled payment system for renal dialysis minus 1 percentage point. However, PPACA amended thisprovision so that the market basket will no longer be subject to a 1 percentage point reduction beginning in 2012, but will be subject to the productivity factor adjustments instead. Beginning in January 1, 2012, providers of renal dialysis services and renal dialysis facilities will be subject to quality incentive requirements and they will be subject to a reduction of up to 2% if they do not meet the requirements.	December 31, 2009 amount, resulting in a composite rate of $135.15 for both hospital-based and independent facilities ser-vices furnished on or after Jan-uary 1, 2010. The drug add-on adjustment for 2010 remained the same as the 2009 adjustment, at $20.33 per treatment. The wage index adjustment for 2010 reflects the latest available wagedate, including a revised budget neutrality adjustment of 1.057888. The ESRD wage index floor was reduced from .70 to .65.

Table 25. (Continued)

Provider/ service	General payment policy	General update policy	Recent update
	prospective payment system for dialysis services furnished either at a facility or in a patient's home, for services furnished beginning on January 1, 2005. The basic case- mix adjusted system has two components: (1) the composite rate, which covers services, including dialysis; and (2) a drug add-on adjustment for the difference between the payment amounts for separately billable drugs and biologicals and their acquisition costs, as determined by Inspector General Reports. MIPPA changed payments for dialysis. Beginning January 1, 2009, the payment rate for dialysis services are "site neutral" and in applying the geographic index to providers of services, the labor share is based on the labor share otherwise applied for renal dialysis facilities. Adjustments are no longer made to the composite rate for hospital-based dialysis facilities to reflect higher overhead costs. MIPPA		

Table 25. (Continued)

Provider/ service	General payment policy	General update policy	Recent update
	requires the Secretary to implement a bundled payment system, making a single payment for Medicare renal dialysis services, beginning January 1, 2011. The bundled payment will include items and services which were included in the composite rate as of December 31, 2010, erythropoiesis stimulating agents (ESAs) and other drugs and biologicals paid for separately (before bundling), and diagnostic laboratory tests among other items. It will not include vaccines. Payments will include adjustments for case mix, high cost outliers (including variations in the amount of ESAs), and costs in rural, low-volume facilities (with a minimum payment adjustment of 10% for services furnished between January 1, 2011, and January 1, 2014), among others. The bundled payments system will be phased-in equally (and budget neutrally) over four years. It will be fully implemented by January 1, 2014.		

Table 26. Managed Care Organizations

Provider/ service	General payment policy	General update policy	Recent update
(a) Medicare advantage contracts	In general, Medicare makes a monthly payment in advance to participating Medicare Advantage (MA) health plans for each enrolled beneficiary in a payment area. In exchange, the plans agree to furnish all Medicare-covered items and services (except hospice) to each enrollee. In general, the actuarial value of basic cost sharing may not exceed the actuarial value of cost sharing under original Medicare. Congress made substantial changes to the Medicare+Choice program with the passage of the MMA in 2003. The act created the Medicare Advantage (MA) program, which replaced the M+C program and introduced several changes designed to increase the availability of private plans for Medicare beneficiaries. In	The MA payments are determined annually by the method described under "General Payment Policy." For CY2004 through CY2009, plan benchmarks were updated annually by the minimum percentage increase, or in certain years, 100% of FFS spending in the area (the rebased amount). The minimum percentage increase is the prior year's benchmark increased by the national MA growth percentage (projected increase in *Medicare per capita expenditures).* In years when the Secretary rebases rates, the benchmark for each county was updated by the greater of either the national MA growth percentage, or 100% of FFS spending adjusted to exclude the	For **CY2009**, MA benchmarks were updated by the greater of either 100% FFS spending, or the previous year's benchmark increased by the national MA growth percentage (4.24%) adjusted for budget neutrality (1.009)—an increase of 3.6%. For **CY2010**, MA benchmarks were not rebased. All bench-marks were updated by the increase in the national MA growth percentage (0.81%), adjusted for budget neutrality (1.001), and the phase-out of indirect medical education (a maximum reduction of approximately 0.6%). Also for CY2010, a uniform 3.4% reduction will be applied to the risk scores of all MA

Table 26. (Continued)

Provider/ service	General payment policy	General update policy	Recent update
	addition to the immediate payment increases to plans, beginning in 2006 the MA program changed the payment structure and introduced regional plans that operate like Preferred Provider Organizations. Additionally, beneficia-ries had access to a drug plan whetherthey were enrolled in original Medicare or a private plan. In 2006, the Secretary began determining MA plan payments by comparing plan bids to a benchmark. A plan's bid is its estimated revenue requirement of providing Part A and B Medicare services to beneficiaries (including cost of services, administration, and profit). A benchmark is the maximum amount CMS will pay a plan for providing these required benefits. If a plan's bid is less than the benchmark, its payment is equal to its bid plus a rebate equal to a percentage of the	value of Medicare direct medical education payments, as explained below. Beginning in 2004 and at a minimum every third year, the Secretary is required to rebase FFS payment rates. Rebasing is updating FFS rates to reflect recent growth in county health care expenditures. The update to the benchmark for regional plans has both a statutory increase and a competitive increase. The statutory component is similar to the update for other MA plans and the competitive component is based on a weighted average of plan bids. DRA made additional changes to the benchmark calculation. Beginning in 2007, DRA added two new adjustments to calculating the benchmark: (1) an adjustment to exclude bud-get neutrality in risk adjustment, and	plan enrollees to account for differences in coding patterns between MA plans and providers under Parts A and B of original Medicare.

Table 26. (Continued)

Provider/ service	General payment policy	General update policy	Recent update
	difference between its bid and the benchmark. (Before 2012, the rebate is equal to 75%; starting in 2012, the size of the rebate is contingent of plan quality, as explained below.) The remaining amount is retained by the federal government. If a plan's bid is greater than the benchmark, its payment is equal to the benchmark amount and the plan must make up the difference between its bid and the benchmark by charging a beneficiary premium. In general, the Secretary has the authority to review and negotiate plan bid amounts to ensure that the bid reflects revenue requirements. At least one plan offered by an MA organization must be an MA-PD plan, one that offers Part D prescription drug coverage. MA organizations offering prescription drug coverage receive a direct subsidy for each enrollee in their MA-PD plan, equal to the	(2) an adjustment to account for coding intensity differences between MA plans and original Medicare for years 2007 through 2010. For purposes of calculating the phase-out of budget neutrality in risk adjustment, the Secretary was required to conduct a study of the difference between treat-ment and coding patterns between MA plans and providers under Parts A and B of Medicare. The findings were to be incor-porated into calculations of MA benchmarks in 2008, 2009, and 2010, however they were first incorporated in 2010. Beginning in 2010, MIPPA requires that the value of indirect medical education be phased-out of all benchmarks. The amount phased-out each year will be based on a ratio of (1) a specified percentage (0.60% in the first	

Table 26. (Continued)

Provider/ service	General payment policy	General update policy	Recent update
	plan's risk adjusted standardized bid amount (reduced by the base beneficiary premium). The plans also receive a reinsurance payment amount for the federal share of their payment as well as premium and cost-sharing reimbursements for qualified low-income enrollees. Also beginning in 2006, the MA program began offering regional planscovering both in- and out-of-network required Medicare services. To encourage regional plan participation in the program additional payments were authorized in certain circumstances for hospitals that would not otherwise join a private plan's network. Beginning in 2012, for MA plans that bid below the benchmark, the rebate will be contingent on plan quality as measured by a 5-star quality rating system established by the Secretary. The calculation will be	year), relative to (2) the proportion of per capita costs in original Medicare in the county that IME costs represent. The effect of the ratio is to phase-out a higher proportion of IME costs in areas where IME makes up a smaller percentage of per capita spending in original Medicare. After 2010, the numerator of the phase-out percentage will be increased by 0.60 percentage points each year. CY2011 benchmarks will be frozen at the CY2010 level. Starting in CY2012, benchmarks will begin to be calculated as a percent of a base rate. In CY2012, the base rate will equal 100% FFS spending in the area and will be updated each year. County benchmarks will be set at either 95%, 100%, 107.5% or 115% of the base rate, with higher	

Table 26. (Continued)

Provider/ service	General payment policy	General update policy	Recent update
	phased in over three years from 75% for all MA plans that bid below the benchmark for years prior to 2012, to a rate of 70% for plans with a star rating of 4.5 or higher, 65% for plans with a star rating of 3.5 or greater, but below 4.5 stars, and 50% for plans with less than 3.5 stars. The rebate based on plan quality will be fully phased-in by 2014.	percentages applied to counties with the lowest FFS spending. The phase-in will take place over 2 to 6 years, with a larger phase-in period for areas where the new methodology would result in larger benchmark decreases. The yearly update to the base rate will either be a rebased amount for all counties, or an increase above the previous years' base equal to the national MA growth percentage for all counties. Also starting in CY2012, benchmarks will be increased based on plan quality with higher increases in qualifying areas. The coding intensity adjustment first specified in DRA will continue after CY2010 with specified minimum adjustments starting in CY2014.	
(b) Cost contracts	Medicare pays cost contract health maintenance organizations (HMOs) and competitive medical plans	No specific update. Cost-based HMOs are paid 100% of their actual costs.	No specific update.

Table 26. (Continued)

Provider/ service	General payment policy	General update policy	Recent update
	(CMPs) the actual costs they incur for furnishing Medicare-covered services (less the estimated value of required Medicare cost sharing), subject to a test of "reasonableness." Interim payment is made to the HMO/CMP on a monthly per capita basis; final payment reconciles interim payments to actual costs. Beginning January 1, 2013, cost contracts can not be extended or renewed in a service area if, during the entire previous year, the service area had two or more MA regional plans or two or more MA local plans offered by different organizations.		

Table 27. Outpatient Prescription Drug Coverage

Provider/ service	General payment policy	General update policy	Recent update
Part D drug coverage. Outpatient prescription drug coverage is provided through private prescription drug plans (PDPs) or MA prescription drug (MA-PD) plans. The program relies on these private plans to provide coverage and to bear some of the financial risk for drug costs; federal subsidies cover the bulk of the risk. Unlike other Medicare services, the benefits can only be obtained through private plans. While all plans have to meet certain minimum requirements, there are significant	Federal payments to plans are linked to "standard coverage." Qualified Part D plans are required to offer either "standard coverage" or alternative coverage, with at least actuarially equivalent benefits. For 2010, most plans offer actuarially equivalent benefits or enhanced coverage rather than the standard package A number of plans have reduced or eliminated the deductible. Many plans offer tiered cost sharing under which lower cost sharing applies for generic drugs, higher cost sharing applies for preferred brand name drugs, and even higher cost sharing applies for non-preferred brand name drugs. Some plans provide some	The definition of standard coverage is updated annually based on the estimated increase in per capita costs for the 12 month period ending the previous July.	In **CY2010**, "standard coverage" has a $310 deductible and 25% coinsurance for costs between $310 and $2,830 (the initial coverage period). From this point, there is no coverage, except for a $250 Medicare rebate mandated by recent legislation, until the beneficiary has out-of-pocket costs of $4,550 ($6,440 in total spending); this coverage gap has been labeled the "doughnut hole." Once the beneficiary reaches the catastrophic limit, the program pays all costs

Table 27. (Continued)

Provider/ service	General payment policy	General update policy	Recent update
differences among them in terms of benefit design, benefici-ary premiums amounts, drugs included on plan formularies (i.e. list of covered drugs) and cost sharing applicable for particular drugs. Drug prices under Part D are determined through negotiations between the PDPs, or MA-PDs, and drug manufacturers. The Secretary of Health and Human Services is statutorily prohibited from intervening in Part D drug price negotiations.	coverage in the coverage gap ("doughnut hole"); this is generally limited to generic drugs.		except for nominal cost sharing. PPACA, as amended by HCERA, mandates phasing out the Part D doughnut hole. Beginning in 2011, manufacurers will be required to provide a 50%discount on brand-name drugs to partici-ate in the Part D program. The law phases in Medicare cove-age for generic drugs during the coverage gap starting in 2011, and for brand name drugs in 2013. When the doughnut hole is fully phased out in 2020, Part D enrollees will be responsible for 25% of the cost of brand name and generic drugs during the cove-age gap

Table 27. (Continued)

Provider/ service	General payment policy	General update policy	Recent update
			(the same as in the initial coverage phase). The catastrophic coverage limit will also be reduced to a small extent in years 2014 through 2019.
Federal Subsidy Payments	Federal subsidy payments (including both direct payments and reinsurance payments) are made to plans consistent with an overall subsidy level of 74.5% for basic coverage. Direct monthly per capita payments are made to a plan equal to the plan's standardized bid amount adjusted for health status and risk and reduced by the base beneficiary premium, as adjusted to reflect the difference between the bid and the national average bid. Reinsurance payments, equal to 80% of allowable costs, are provided for enrollees whose costs exceed the annual out-of-pocket threshold ($4,550 in 2010).	Payments to plans are calculated annually by the method described under "General Payment Policy."	Federal payments were recalculated for the 2010 plan year.

Table 27. (Continued)

Provider/ service	General payment policy	General update policy	Recent update
Beneficiary Premiums	Beneficiary premiums represent on average 25.5% of the cost of the basic benefit. A base beneficiary premium is calculated based on the national average monthly bid amount for basic coverage. This amount is then adjusted, up or down as appropriate, to reflect differences between the plan's standardized bid amount and the national average monthly bid amount. It is further increased for any supplemental benefits and decreased if the individual is entitled to a low-income subsidy. The premium is the same for all individuals in a particular plan	Beneficiary premiums are calculated annually by the method described under "General Payment Policy."	Beneficiary premiums were recalculated for the 2010 plan year. The base beneficiary premium for 2010 is $31.94. (Actual premiums paid by individual beneficiaries vary from one Part D plan to another.)
Risk corridors	The federal government and plans share the risk for costs within specified "risk corridors."Risk corridors" are specified percentages for costs above and below a target amount; the target amount is defined as total	In 2006 and 2007, plans were at full risk for costs within 2.5% above or below the target. If costs were between 2.5% and 5% above the target, they were at risk for 25% of spending between 2.5% and	The 2010 risk corridors are modified, as described under "General Update Policy."

Table 27. (Continued)

Provider/ service	General payment policy	General update policy	Recent update
	payments paid to the plan taking into account the amount paid to the plan by the government and enrollees.	5% of the target and 20% of spending above that amount. If plans fell Below the target, they have to refund 75% of the savings if costs fall between 2.5% and 5% below the target and 80% of any amounts below 5% of the target. For 2008-2011, risk corridors are modified. Plans are at full risk for spending within 5% above or below the target. They are at risk for 50% of spending between 5% and 10% of the target and 20% of any spending exceeding 10% of the target.	

End Notes

[1] Certain non-physicians providers (such as physician assistants, nurse practitioners, clinical nurse specialists, certified nurse midwives, psychologists, and social workers) are permitted to furnish services and bill Medicare under the physician fees schedule (PFS). In this report, the term "physician" or "practitioner" will include all such providers unless otherwise specified.

[2] Not all services require cost sharing from a beneficiary. For instance, clinical laboratory services and home health services under Parts A and B of Medicare do not require payments from a beneficiary or a beneficiary's insurance, such as Medicare supplemental insurance (Medigap), Medicaid, or employer-sponsored retiree health insurance. Cost- sharing requirements under Part C plans may differ from those under Parts A and B for the same service.

[3] For more information, see CRS Report RL3 1223, *Medicare: Supplementary "Medigap" Coverage*.

[4] The MMA required the Secretary to establish and implement a competitive bidding program for durable medical equipment, prosthetics, orthotics and certain supplies. The program would pay for certain items based on the bids of qualified suppliers in designated areas. The first round of the competitive bidding program started July 1, 2008. However, MIPPA stopped the program, terminated all contracts with suppliers, and required the Secretary to rebid the first round in 2009. Expansion of the program was delayed by two years until 2011. See CRS Report R4121 1, *Medicare Durable Medical Equipment: The Competitive Bidding Program*.

[5] For details, see CRS Report R40907, *Medicare Physician Payment Updates and the Sustainable Growth Rate (SGR) System*.

[6] In 2010, for each spell of illness, a beneficiary deductible is $1,100 to cover day 1 through 60 in a hospital. The daily coinsurance charge is $275 for each day from 61 through 90. After 90 days in the hospital, a beneficiary may draw down 60 lifetime reserve days with a daily coinsurance of $550.

[7] Generally, Part B premiums are set to cover 25% of the actuarial cost of Part B services for an aged beneficiary. Income-related Part B premiums were introduced by the Medicare Modernization Act (P.L. 108-173) and first took effect in 2007. For more information, see CRS Report R40082, *Medicare: Part B Premiums* and CRS Report R40561, *The Effect of No Social Security COLA on Medicare Part B Premiums*.

[8] Through 2005, managed care plans had the option to charge a premium for basic part A and B Medicare benefits only if the value of cost sharing for basic benefits was reduced by the same amount. If a plan chose to offer supplemental benefits not covered under original Medicare, the plan could charge a supplemental premium equal to the actuarial value of supplemental benefits; the value of the supplemental premium was not constrained by cost-sharing levels for basic Medicare benefits. All beneficiaries in Part C and original Medicare are required to pay a Part B premium, unless the Part C plan pays-down the value of the Part B premium as part of a supplemental benefit.

[9] Plans must also adhere to specific constraints on enrollee cost-sharing. Beginning in 2011, cost sharing under an MA plan may not exceed that under original Medicare for certain services, such as chemotherapy treatment, renal dialysis, skilled nursing care and other services identified by the Secretary.

[10] For a general discussion on productivity measurement and growth, see CRS Report RL34677, *Productivity Growth: Trends and Prospects*. For a detailed description of the productivity adjustment as it applies to Medicare FFS providers, see CRS Report R41 196, *Medicare Provisions in the Patient Protection and Affordable Care Act (PPACA): Summary and Timeline*.

[11] The Balanced Budget Act of 1997 first introduced the concept of productivity adjusted payment increases for physician services, however, Congress has overwritten the effects of the productivity adjustment in recent years. For more information, see CRS Report R40907, *Medicare Physician Payment Updates and the Sustainable Growth Rate (SGR) System*.

[12] The Boards of Trustees, Federal Hospital Insurance and Federal Supplementary Medical Insurance Trust Funds, "2010 Annual Report," August 5, 2010, http://www.cms.gov/ReportsTrustFunds/downloads/tr2010.pdf.

[13] For more information, see CRS Report 97-802, *Medicare Provisions in the Balanced Budget Act of 1997 (BBA 97, P.L. 105-33)*.

[14] For more information, see CRS Report RL3 0347, *Medicare: Changes to Balanced Budget Act of 1997 (BBA 97, P.L. 105-33) Provisions*.

[15] For more information, see CRS Report RL3 0707, *Medicare Provisions in the Medicare, Medicaid, and SCHIP Benefits Improvement and Protection Act of 2000 (BIPA, P.L. 106-554)*.

[16] For more information, see CRS Report RL3 1966, *Overview of the Medicare Prescription Drug, Improvement, and Modernization Act of 2003*.

[17] For more information, see CRS Report RL33251, *Side-by-Side Comparison of Medicare, Medicaid, and SCHIP Provisions in the Deficit Reduction Act of 2005*.

[18] For more information, see CRS Report RL34360, *P.L. 110-173: Provisions in the Medicare, Medicaid, and SCHIP Extension Act of 2007*.

[19] For more information, see CRS Report RL34592, *P.L. 110-275: The Medicare Improvements for Patients and Providers Act of 2008*.

[20] For more information, see CRS Report R41 196, *Medicare Provisions in the Patient Protection and Affordable Care Act (PPACA): Summary and Timeline*.

In: Medicare Payment Policies and Issues
Editors: Alexander D. Hoffmann
ISBN: 978-1-61122-896-0

Chapter 2

MEDICARE PHYSICIAN PAYMENT UPDATES AND THE SUSTAINABLE GROWTH RATE (SGR) SYSTEM

Jim Hahn

SUMMARY

Each year since 2002, the statutory method for determining the annual updates to the Medicare physician fee schedule, known as the sustainable growth rate (SGR) system, has resulted in a reduction in the reimbursement rates (or a "negative update"). With the exception of 2002, when a 4.8% decrease was applied, Congress has passed a series of bills to override the reductions. The SGR system was established because of the concern that the Medicare fee schedule itself would not adequately constrain overall increases in spending for physicians' services. While the fee schedule limits the amount that Medicare will pay for each service, there are no limits on the volume or mix of services. The SGR system was intended to serve as a restraint on aggregate spending. If expenditures over a period are less than the cumulative spending target for the period, the update is increased. However, if spending exceeds the cumulative spending target over a certain period, future updates are reduced to bring spending back in line with the target.

In the first few years of the SGR system, the actual expenditures did not exceed the targets and the updates to the physician fee schedule were close to the Medicare economic index (MEI, a price index of inputs required to produce physician services) in the first two years (2.3% in 1998 and 1999, compared with a MEI of 2.2% in 1998 and 2.3% in 1999). For the next two years, in 2000 and 2001, the actual physician fee schedule update was more than twice the MEI for those years (5.5% update vs. MEI of 2.4% in 2000, 5.0% update vs. MEI of 2.1% in 2001). However, beginning in 2002, the actual expenditure exceeded allowed targets and the discrepancy has grown with each year, resulting in a series of ever-larger cuts under the formula.

Some criticisms of the SGR system point to purported flaws in the technical details behind the formula, while others have just expressed displeasure with the resultant outcome. Although modifications have been proposed to replace the SGR system, no proposal has garnered sufficient support and almost all proposals would be expensive to implement compared against the current baseline, which necessarily assumes that significant cuts to the fee schedule will occur.

Legislative activity in the current session of Congress includes several bills. The FY2010 Defense Appropriations Act delayed the implementation of the reductions for two months, through February 28, 2010. The Statutory Pay-As-You-Go Act of 2010 (P.L. 111-139) exempts the amount it would cost to freeze payments for five years from PAYGO rules. H.R. 4691, which became law on March 2, 2010, delayed the payment cuts through March 31, 2010. On April 15, the Senate passed an amended version of H.R. 4851 that extended the payment cut delay through May 31, 2010. The House passed the amended bill, and the President signed P.L. 111-157 into law that day. On June 25, 2010, several weeks after the expiration of the extension created by the Continuing Extension Act, an amended version of H.R. 3962 was signed into law that increases fee schedule payments 2.2% retroactive to June 1 and continuing through November 30, 2010.

INTRODUCTION

Each year since 2002, the statutory method for determining the annual updates to the Medicare physician fee schedule, known as the sustainable growth rate (SGR) system, has resulted in a reduction in the reimbursement rates (or a "negative update").[1] With the exception of 2002, when a 4.8% decrease was applied, Congress has passed a series of bills to override the reductions. However, these actions have required almost yearly attention from the Congress. This report provides a background on the Medicare fee schedule, the SGR system and the annual updates, and discusses recent proposals to address this issue.

Background on the Medicare Fee Schedule Updates

Medicare payments for Part B services[2] provided by physicians and certain non-physician practitioners are made on the basis of a fee schedule, a list of over 7,000 tasks and services for which physicians bill Medicare.[3] From the inception of the program until 1992 and the introduction of the resource-based relative value scale (RB-RVS) fee schedule, Medicare paid physicians based on "usual, customary, and reasonable" charges.[4]

The Omnibus Budget Reconciliation Act (OBRA 89, P.L. 101-239) created the RB-RVS-based Medicare fee schedule, which went into effect January 1, 1992. Under the RB-RVS fee schedule, the Center for Medicare and Medicaid Services (CMS) assigns relative values that reflect physician work (i.e., time, skill, and intensity it takes to provide the service), practice expenses, and malpractice costs.[5] The adjusted relative values are then multiplied by a conversion factor to derive the actual payment amount in dollars. Medicare pays providers the lesser of the actual charge for the service or the allowed amount under the fee schedule.

Updates and the Sustainable Growth Rate (SGR) System

The SGR system was established because of the concern that the Medicare fee schedule itself would not adequately constrain overall increases in spending for physicians' services. While the fee schedule limits the amount that Medicare will pay for each service, there are no limits on the volume or mix of services. The SGR system was intended to serve as a restraint on aggregate spending. While the SGR targets are not limits on expenditures, they represent a "sustainable" trajectory for cumulative spending on Medicare physician services from April 1996 forward. The annual fee schedule update thus reflects the success or failure in meeting the goal. If expenditures over a period are less than the cumulative spending target for the period, the update is increased. However, if spending exceeds the cumulative spending target over a certain period, the update for a future year is reduced, with the goal to bring spending back in line with the target.

Expenditure targets have been a factor in the calculation of Medicare physician payment updates since the current fee schedule was first implemented in 1992. In the first year, one overall conversion factor was used to calculated the update. Then, two (surgical and non-surgical services) and eventually three conversion factors were used for different categories of services (surgical, primary care, and other nonsurgical services). However, under the Medicare Volume Performance Standard (MVPS) method, targets were set (and typically exceeded) each year; there was no cumulative goal and no significant consequence to exceeding the expenditure target. The current SGR method for calculating annual updates was created partly in response to the shortcomings of the prior method.

The Balanced Budget Act of 1997 (BBA97, P.L. 105-33) replaced the MVPS with the SGR, with the objective of creating a *sustainable* growth path for Part B expenditures. First, BBA97 added a cumulative spending criteria that resulted in actual consequences for failing to meet expenditure targets; beginning with April 1, 1996, as the starting point, actual program expenditures are compared to growth targets to determine annual updates. Second, BBA 97 introduced the rate of growth in the per capita amount of the gross domestic product (GDP) into the SGR calculation and also provided for the use of a single conversion factor instead of three.[6] By tying the expenditure targets to the growth in GDP per capita, this system attempted to hold Medicare physician expenditures to a level that would not consume an ever-increasing share of national income.

Since the conversion factor applies to all services, the update to the conversion factor is the key component for determining how reimbursements change from year to year.

Conversion Factor Calculation

The annual update to the conversion factor calculation is based on (1) the Medicare Economic Index (MEI), which measures the weighted average annual price changes in the inputs needed to produce physician services;[7] (2) the Update Adjustment Factor (UAF), used to equate actual and target (allowed) expenditures; and (3) allowed expenditures, equal to the actual expenditures updated by the SGR.

Sustainable Growth Rate (SGR)

The SGR sets both the cumulative and allowed expenditures under the UAF formula and consists of the following components:

- the estimated percentage changes in physicians fees,
- the estimated percentage changes in the number of fee-for-service beneficiaries,
- the estimated percentage growth in real gross domestic product (GDP) per capita (10-year moving average), and
- the estimated percentage changes resulting from changes in laws and regulations.

One important implication of the way this formula was constructed is that sustainable growth in Medicare physician expenditures should be equivalent to the rate of growth in the economy (i.e., the growth in GDP per capita). In addition, the formula implies that increases in managed care enrollment relative to fee-for-service Medicare would result in a slightly lower SGR.

Update Adjustment Factor

The update adjustment sets the conversion factor at a level so that projected spending for the year will meet allowed spending by the end of the year. The adjustment factor is the sum of (1) the prior year adjustment component; and (2) the cumulative adjustment component. Use of both the prior year adjustment component and the cumulative adjustment component allows any deviation between cumulative actual expenditures and cumulative allowed expenditures to be corrected over several years rather than a single year. As originally established, the adjustment factor can not be less than minus 7% or more than plus 3%. Thus, despite calculations which would have led to larger reductions, the UAF adjustment has been minus 7% for the last several years. The caps on the adjustment limit the annual reduction or increase. Thus, the gap between cumulative actual spending and cumulative allowed spending grows larger each year and is exacerbated whenever Congress overrides the reductions, since the targets are never modified under current law.

HISTORICAL UPDATES AND LEGISLATIVE OVERRIDES

Under the update formula, if actual expenditures do not exceed target expenditures, the update generally would be positive and payments would increase for all services under the fee schedule subject to the single conversion factor. In the first few years of the SGR system, the actual expenditures did not exceed the targets. (See **Figure 1**.) As a consequence, the updates to the physician fee schedule were close to the MEI in the first two years (2.3% in 1998 and 1999, compared with MEI of 2.2% in 1998 and 2.3% in 1999).[8] For the next two years, in 2000 and 2001, the actual physician fee schedule update was more than twice the MEI for those years (5.5% update vs. MEI of 2.4% in 2000, 5.0% update vs. MEI of 2.1% in 2001). However, beginning in 2002, the actual expenditure exceeded allowed targets and the discrepancy has grown with each year.

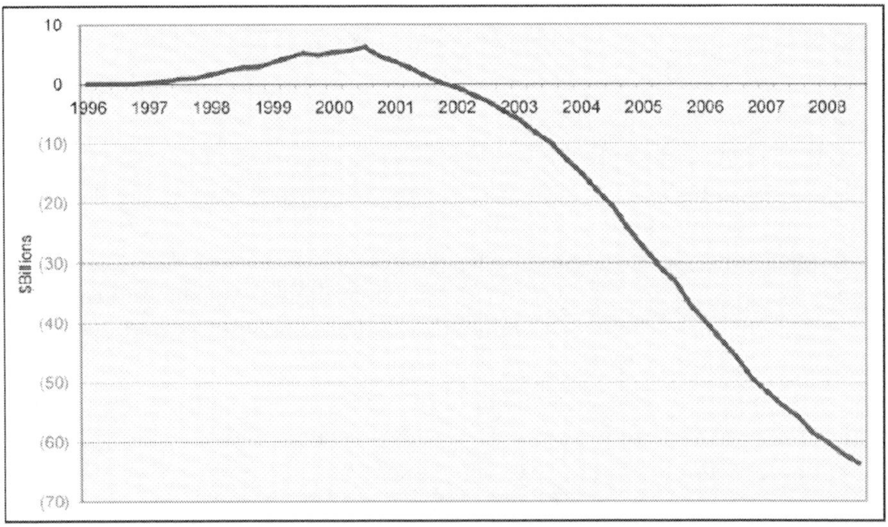

Source: CRS figure from CMS data contained in "Estimated Sustainable Growth Rate and Conversion Factor, for Medicare Payments to Physicians in 2010." Available at http://www.cms.hhs.gov/SustainableGRatesConFact/ Downloads/sgr2010p.pdf

Notes: This graph shows the difference between *cumulative* allowed expenditures and actual expenditures for physician services. The 2008 figures for both allowed and actual expenditures are CMS estimates.

Figure 1. Difference Between Cumulative Allowed and Actual Expenditures for Physician Services Under the SGR System 1996-2008

Table 1. Summary of Updates and Legislative Activity 2002-2009

Year	Formula update	Actual update	Legislation	Notes
2002	-4.8%	-4.8%		
2003	-4.4%	1.4%	Consolidated Appropriations Resolution of 2003 (CAR)	The update was 1.7% but was effective on March 1, 2003, so the average update for the year was 1.4%.
2004	-4.5%	1.5%	Medicare Modernization Act of 2003 (MMA, P.L. 108-173)	
2005	-3.3%	1.5%	MMA	
2006	-4.4%	0.2%	Deficit Reduction Act of 2005 (DRA, P.L. 109-171)	Although the DRA froze the conversion factor update, refinements to the RVUs resulted in a 0.2% update for the year.
2007	-5.0%	0%	Tax Relief and Health Care Act of 2006 (TRHCA, P.L. 109-432)	
Jan-Jun 2008	-10.1%	0.5%	Medicare, Medicaid, and SCHIP Extension Act of 2007 (MMSEA, P.L. 110-173)	Physicians who voluntarily reported on certain quality measures during July 1, 2007-December 31, 2007, were eligible for a bonus payment of 1.5% in 2008 per TRHCA.
Jul-Dec 2008	-10.6% reduction from June 2008 level	0% (0.5% from 2007 level)	Medicare Improvement for Patients and Providers Act of 2008 (MIPPA, P.L. 110-275)	See above.
2009		1.1%	MIPPA	Physicians who voluntarily reported on certain quality measures during 2008 were eligible for a bonus payment of 1.5% in 2009 per MMSEA.

Table 1. (Continued)

Year	Formula update	Actual update	Legislation	Notes
Jan 1-Feb 28, 2010	-21.3%	0%	Department of Defense Appropriations Act (P.L. 111-118)	
Mar 1-Mar 31, 2010		0%	Temporary Extension Act (P.L. 111-144)	Signed into law on Mar 2, 2010.
Apr 1-May 31, 2010		0%	Continuing Extension Act (P.L. 111-157)	Signed into law on Apr 15, 2010.
June 1-November 30, 2010		2.2%	Preservation of Access to Care for Medicare Beneficiaries and Pension Relief Act of 2010 (P.L. 111-192)	Signed into law on June 25, 2010. (increase was retroactive to June 1.)

Source: 2010 Annual Report of the Boards of Trustees of the Federal Hospital Insurance And Federal Supplementary Medical Insurance Trust Funds, http://www.cms.hhs.gov/ReportsTrustFunds/downloads/ tr2010.pdf, and CMS, Estimated Sustainable Growth Rate and Conversion Factor, for Medicare Payments to Physicians in 2011, http://www.cms.hhs.gov/Sustainable GRates Con Fact/Downloads/sgr2011p.pdf.

As a consequence of exceeding the target, the formula dictated a reduction in the fee schedule in 2002. Although reductions have been called for every year since, Congress has passed legislation that has overridden the cuts each year since. (See **Table 1**.)

In addition to overriding the payment reductions, Congress has also included provisions in several of the laws to increase Medicare physician payments in other ways. For example, the Congress has altered the geographic adjustment factor for physician work, one component used in making regional adjustments to payments under the physician fee schedule. MMA set a floor on the work geographic adjustment index at 1.0 for 2004-2006, thereby slightly increasing the payment amounts in some areas. TRHCA extended this provision through 2007, MMSEA extended it through June 30, 2008, and MIPPA extends it through December 2009. In addition, beginning January 1, 2009, MIPPA also raised the work geographic adjustment in Alaska to 1.5.

Some of the bills also modified the cap on the conversion factor, which has led to the current situation where the consequence of not overriding the reduction would lead to cuts in excess of the 7% cap. TRHCA specified that the override of the reduction that would have been implemented under the statutory formula was to be treated as if it did not occur. Therefore, the starting base for the 2008 calculation was 5% below the actual 2007 conversion factor. MMSEA overrode the reduction for the first six months of 2008 and provided for a 0.5% increase for that period. However, the legislation again specified that the override of the statutory formula was to be treated as if it did not occur. MIPPA again specified that the override of the statutory formula was to be treated as if it did not occur. As a result, CMS estimates that a reduction of 21.2% will be necessary in 2010 unless Congress acts again to override the current situation.[9]

Analysis and Criticisms of SGR System

The experience in recent years has been that the volume and the intensity of physician services provided to Medicare beneficiaries are growing at more than double the rate allowed under the SGR system.[10] Payment reductions as called for under the update formula have required almost annual interventions by Congress and the SGR system has been criticized (and defended) amid calls for its repeal. While some of the criticisms of the SGR system point to purported flaws in the technical details behind the formula, others have just expressed general displeasure with the outcome.

General and Conceptual Concerns

One commonly asserted criticism is that the SGR system treats all services and physicians equally in the calculation of the annual payment update to the detriment of physicians who are "unduly" penalized. The expenditure target is a nationwide aggregate and the annual updates are applied uniformly; there is no direct link between individual behavior and the subsequent update. Thus, actions might be individually rational (physicians provide and bill for additional services and collect greater reimbursement) yet collectively detrimental (the annual update is reduced).[11] An individual physician who controls or reduces volume does not see a resulting increase in payments.

Others point out that there is no ability to distinguish between appropriate volume increases (for instance, due to changes in disease conditions that increase demand) and inappropriate volume increases (for instance, when tests or procedures are provided that are not necessary).

Technical Concerns

The inclusion of some items and services in the expenditure targets has also been called into question. Specifically, physicians have argued that Part B drug spending should be excluded from the calculation because physicians have no control or influence on the price of these drugs, although CMS is preparing to address this in its implementation of the 2010 proposed rule changes.[12]

Additionally, the targets may not be not adequately modified to reflect scientific and technological innovations or site-of-service shifts, and providers have often stated that actual increases in practice costs exceed those allowed under the system. The impact of legislative and regulatory changes also may not be fully reflected in the SGR calculation.

Per Capita Gross Domestic Product (GDP) and the Annual Update

The SGR is based on a number of factors, including the changes in the price of inputs required to produce physician services (such as rent, staff and supplies), the change in the number of Medicare fee-for-service beneficiaries, the effect of laws and regulations on part B expenditures, and the rate of growth in the per capita gross domestic product, calculated as a 10-year moving average.

The rate of growth in per capita GDP has a significant impact on the determination of the annual update. As can be seen in **Figure 2**, from 1997 through 2000, per capita GDP grew faster than part B expenditures, at more than 4% annually; part B expenditures were relatively stable from 1996 to 1998 and then started to increase in 1999 and 2000. However, economic growth slowed at the turn of the century (as can be seen in the flatter slope in the growth of per capita GDP during the period from 2000-2003), while part B expenditures grew at a faster rate from 2000 on. Because the comparison of actual to target expenditures includes a significant component that is cumulative (rather than just a comparison of the current period), the updates were positive during the early years of the SGR system but then became negative as a result of this imbalance. (See **Figure 3**.)

Thus, the relative health of the economy effectively masked the increases in total part B expenditures for the first few years under the SGR system, but as the economy slowed and expenditures continued to increase, the updates as determined under the SGR system have turned negative in order to bring projected actual expenditures back in line with target expenditures.

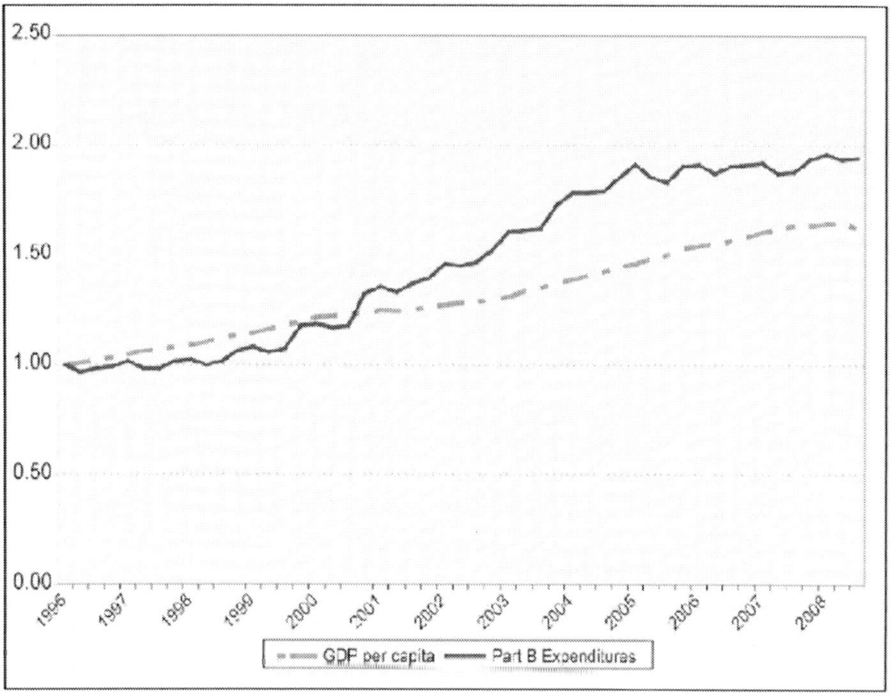

Source: CMS, "Estimated Sustainable Growth Rate and Conversion Factor for Medicare Payments to Physicians in 2010" http://www.cms.hhs.gov/SustainableGRatesConFact/Downloads/sgr2010p.pdf and U.S. Department of Commerce, Bureau of Economic Analysis, *National Income and Product Accounts*, Table 7.1. "Selected Per Capita Product and Income Series in Current and Chained Dollars" (http://www.bea.gov/national/nipaweb/ IndexP.htm#P).

Notes: The lines are based on quarterly data that are not seasonally adjusted. The uneven pattern of Medicare Part B expenditures reflects typical seasonal variation in health care use, which tends to increase with colder temperatures.

Figure 2. Relative Increase in Part B Expenditures vs. per Capita GDP 1996-2008

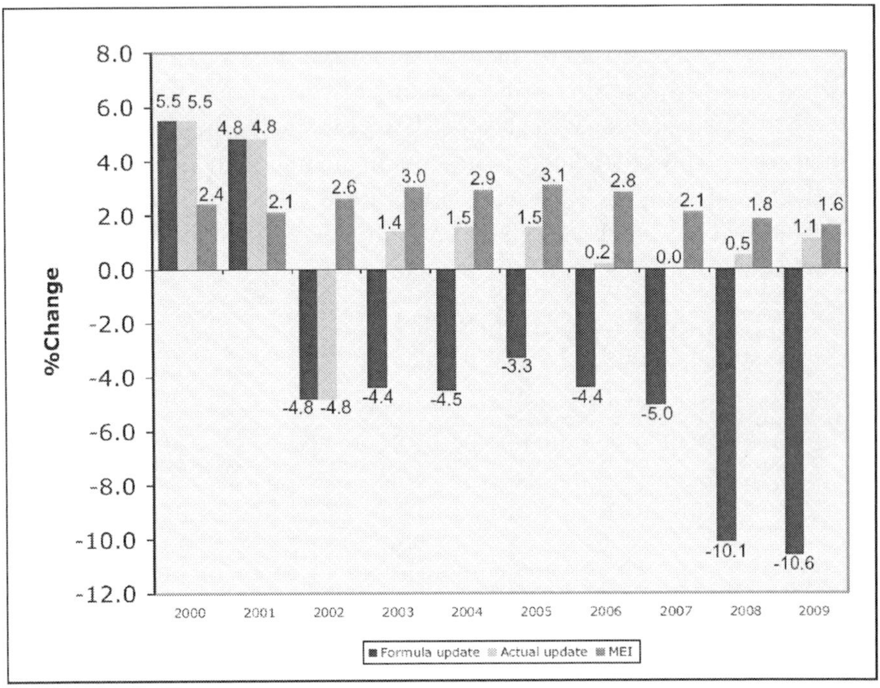

Source: 2009 Annual Report of the Boards of Trustees of the Federal Hospital Insurance And Federal Supplementary Medical Insurance Trust Funds, p. 22. http://www.cms.hhs.gov/ReportsTrustFunds/downloads/ tr2009.pdf, and CMS, Estimated Sustainable Growth Rate and Conversion Factor, for Medicare Payments to Physicians in 2010, http://www.cms.hhs.gov/SustainableGRates ConFact/Downloads/sgr2010p.pdf.

Notes: MMSEA included a six-month override of the SGR update (-10.1%) for the first half of 2008. MIPPA provided for an 18-month override of the SGR update that would have taken effect on July 1, 2008 (-10.6%) that included the second half of 2008 and all of 2009. See also **Table 1**.

Figure 3. Formula Updates, Actual Updates, and the Medicare Economic Index 2000-2009

Potential Modifications and Alternatives

Although a number of modifications to the SGR system have been proposed, there is no consensus around a long-run alternative. In addition, any permanent change would likely be quite costly because the Congressional

Budget Office (CBO) baseline must assume that a reduction in the conversion factor will occur for the next several years as required under current law. In addition to the impact on federal outlays, any change in the update formula will also have implications for beneficiaries; because Part B beneficiary premiums must cover 25% of Part B program costs, any overall increase in spending results in a proportional increase in premiums.[13]

Suggested modifications have ranged from modifying the current formula to replacing the formula and linking updates to payment adequacy and/or quality measures. While a change in the formula would require legislation, some observers have suggested that there are things CMS could do administratively to ease the impact of the current formula. Proponents argue that these changes, such as removing Part B drugs from the calculation, could somewhat moderate the negative updates that are predicted.

The Medicare Modernization Act of 2003 (MMA) required that GAO study "the appropriateness of the sustainable growth rate formula" and "the stability and predictability of such updates and rate and alternatives."[14] In a 2005 report, the GAO categorized options for alternatives around two themes: (1) proposals that end the use of spending targets and separate fee updates from explicit efforts to moderate spending growth; and (2) proposals that retain spending targets but modify the current SGR system to address perceived shortcomings.[15] The first approach emphasizes stable fee updates, while the second automatically adjusts fee updates if spending growth deviates from a predetermined target. GAO stated that "the choice between the two approaches may hinge on whether primary consideration should be given to stable fee increases or to the need for fiscal discipline within the Medicare program." The second approach would end targets as an explicit measure for moderating spending growth. Updates would be based on cost increases with the possibility of specifically addressing high volume service categories such as medical imaging.

The Deficit Reduction Act of 2005 (DRA) required MedPAC to submit a report to Congress on mechanisms that could be used to replace the SGR system, including "such recommendations on alternative mechanisms to replace the sustainable growth rate system as the Medicare Payment Advisory Commission determines appropriate."[16] In its March 2007 report, MedPAC described two possible paths: one path would eliminate the SGR and emphasize the development and adoption of approaches for improving incentives for physicians and other providers to furnish lower cost and higher quality care, while the second path would add a new system of expenditure targets in addition to these approaches.[17] However, MedPAC did not make any recommendations in favor of any single alternative to the SGR, citing "significant disagreement … within the Commission about the utility of expenditure targets" and stating that the complexity of the issues made it difficult to recommend any option with confidence. MedPAC did stress in the report that "a major investment should be made in Medicare's capability to develop, implement, and refine payment systems to reward quality and efficient use of resources while improving payment equity." Examples cited by MedPAC include pay-for-performance programs for quality, improving payment accuracy, and bundling payments to reduce overutilization.

MedPAC has also recommended updating payments for physicians' services based on the estimated change in input prices for the coming year less an adjustment for savings attributable to increased productivity. Specifically, input prices would be measured using the MEI (without regard to the CMS adjustment for productivity increases). The recommended productivity adjustment would be that used across all provider services.[18]

In March 2008, CBO issued cost estimates for a variety of approaches for dealing with the physician payment issue.[19] Proposals with modest costs assumed a freeze for the second half of 2008 (as opposed to a 10.6% reduction), with reductions in future years to hold future rates at current law levels. More costly alternatives would freeze or increase payments over the 10-year budget window. For example, increasing payments by the MEI each year through 2018 would increase federal spending by $288.1 billion for the FY2008-FY2018 period. Coupling this with a provision excluding this change from beneficiary premium calculations ("premium hold-harmless") would increase federal spending by $364.3 billion over the same period.

Figure 3 shows that in each year since 2002, the MEI has been greater than the update as determined under the SGR formula and the actual update that physicians have received as a result of congressional intervention.

Recent Legislative Activity

H.R. 3162 (110th Congress)

Summary

The Children's Health and Medicare Protection Act of 2007 (CHAMP, H.R. 3162) was introduced on July 24, 2007. Section 301 of Title III would have modified the SGR system by eliminating the single conversion factor currently applied to all physician services and would have established separate target growth rates and conversion factors for each of six newly created service categories.[20] The six categories of physician services would have been the following: evaluation and management services for primary care and for preventive services; other evaluation and management services; imaging services and diagnostic tests; major procedures; anesthesia services; and minor procedures and other services.

The provision would have replaced the single SGR computation with separate target growth rates for each of the service categories created above. Beginning with 2008, the target growth rate for each service category would have been computed and applied separately using the same method for computing the sustainable growth rate under current law except that (1) "physicians' services" would refer to the physicians' services included in the appropriate service category, (2) the estimate of the annual average percentage growth in real gross domestic product per capita for the applicable period would have been increased by 0.03, and (3) a national coverage determination would be treated as a change in regulation and thus incorporated into the Secretary's estimate of the percentage change in expenditures for all physicians' services in the fiscal year (compared with the previous fiscal year) resulting from changes in law and regulations.

Beginning with 2008, the conversion factors would be computed and updated separately for each service category. In 2008, the conversion factors would have been based on the single 2007 conversion factor multiplied by the appropriate update for the category. In subsequent years, the conversion factor for each category would have been based on the conversion factor for the service category adjusted by the appropriate update. The provision would have established a floor for updates so that the conversion factors for each service category would be no less than 0.5% for 2008 and 2009.

The Committee on Ways and Means amended and reported the bill on August 1, 2007, and the House passed the bill the same day by a vote of 225-204.[21] The bill was never taken up by the Senate.

Brief Analysis

The approach to modifying the SGR as proposed in H.R. 3162 attempted to address, among other things, the criticism that the current update calculation penalized (or rewarded) all physicians identically regardless of the individual's or the specialty's contribution towards meeting or exceeding the aggregate expenditure target. Thus, even though imaging services have grown faster than other types of physician services (including evaluation and management services, tests, major procedures, and other procedures) the resulting impact on the annual update factor applies to all services across all specialties. However, others have countered that this delineation may not be appropriate and the CHAMP approach went too far. For example, some of the increase in imaging services may have allowed for the earlier detection of disease conditions such as cancer, which may have produced savings for other services and specialties (e.g., nuclear medicine and oncology services).

S. 1776 (111th Congress)

Summary

S. 1776, the Medicare Physician Fairness Act of 2009, was introduced on October 13, 2009. The bill would have (1) set the update to the conversion factor at 0 for 2010 and in subsequent years, and (2) sunset the SGR system immediately. On October 21, 2009, the cloture motion to proceed to the bill was not invoked by the Senate by a vote of 47-53.[22]

Brief Analysis

Setting the update to the conversion factor at 0 would have effectively frozen the Medicare physician fee schedule at 2009 levels in perpetuity, barring other changes. No replacement to the SGR method for determining annual updates was proposed as a substitute. The periodic review of RVUs and the subsequent reallocation of weights would still have affected the relative reimbursements across services, however, because such adjustments are implemented in a budget neutral manner, the physician reimbursements would not have increased overall as a result of this bill.

H.R. 3961 (111th Congress)

Summary

H.R. 3961, the Medicare Physician Payment Reform Act of 2009 was introduced on October 20, 2009. The proposals in this bill share some of the same approaches and objectives as Section 301 of the CHAMP Act, but also differ significantly in a few important ways. First, rather than creating six different categories of physician services, the bill would create two categories of service beginning in 2011, each with its own separate target growth rate and conversion factor update. The two categories of service would be (1) evaluation, management, and preventive services, and (2) all other services. Target expenditures for the E&M and preventive services category would be allowed to grow at the rate of growth of per capita GDP plus 2%, while the target expenditures for the all other category would be allowed to grow at the rate of growth of per capita GDP plus 1%. Second, the year 2009 would be established as the new baseline year for calculating expenditure targets (rather than 1996 under current law) for each of the two categories of services. Third, only physician services would be included in the calculation of actual and target growth expenditures; services provided incident to the physician visit (such as laboratory services), would not be included. Fourth, during the transition to the calculations required for the new method of calculating targets and updates, the 2010 update would be the percentage increase in the Medicare economic index (MEI). In its final rule for 2010 Medicare physician payments, CMS specified that the MEI will be 1.2%.[23]

On November 19, 2009, the House passed H.R. 3961 by a vote of 243-183.[24] However, on February 24, 2010, the Senate amended the bill by replacing everything after the enacting clause and renamed the bill "An Act to extend expiring provisions of the USA PATRIOT Improvement and Reauthorization Act of 2005 and Intelligence Reform and Terrorism Prevention Act of 2004 until February 28, 2011."[25]

Brief Analysis

The impact of this bill would be felt not only by physicians but also by other parts of the Medicare program, the Department of Defense TRICARE program, and beneficiaries under Medicare Part B. CBO estimates that enacting H.R. 3961 would increase direct spending by about $210 billion over the 2010-2019 period.[26] Not only would physician reimbursements under the Medicare physician fee schedule increase, but expenditures under the Medicare Advantage (MA) program would increase because per beneficiary spending for fee-for-service beneficiaries would increase as a result of the bill, raising the "benchmarks" that Medicare uses to determine the capitation payments for beneficiaries enrolled in Medicare Advantage plans. TRICARE expenditures would rise because its physician reimbursements are based on Medicare's physician fee schedule. Furthermore, since Medicare Part B beneficiary premiums are required to cover 25% of total Part B expenditures, the increases in physician reimbursements as a result of changing the update calculation would put pressure on future Part B premiums to rise.

The proposed modification might reduce the likelihood that future expenditures exceed the target expenditures, since the growth rates would be more generous under this bill than under current law, but this might lead to an increase in the total expenditures of the Medicare Part B program. While the SGR has been heavily criticized, a fundamental assumption was that tying physician expenditure growth to the rate of growth in GDP per capita could lead to a sustainable growth path. By allowing the two categories to grow at GDP per capita plus 1% or 2%, this bill would appear to allow for a situation where physician expenditures grow and consume a greater percentage of the national income.

A Senate Amendment in the form of a Substitute to H.R. 3590 (111th Congress)

Summary

Section 3101 of the Senate health care reform bill, an amendment in the form of a substitute to H.R. 3590, would have overridden the reduction in the annual update to the conversion factor used in the determination of the Medicare fee schedule and provided an increase of 0.5% in 2010. The conversion factor for 2011 and for subsequent years would have been computed as if the increase in 2010 had never applied. CBO estimates that this provision would have cost $7.2 billion in 2010 and $4.1 billion in 2011, with no other budgetary impact in subsequent years. However, the manager's amendment contained several additions and modifications to the bill, including Section 10310, which repealed Section 3101. On December 24, 2009, the Senate passed the amended bill by a vote of 60-39.[27]

Brief Analysis

Much as other recent overrides have done, the original provision (Section 3101) would have increased Medicare physician payments slightly in the short term while increasing the cost of addressing this problem in the future because another year's worth of actual expenditures that exceed target expenditures would have contributed to the total amounts that would have to be recouped under the current SGR system. However, the manager's amendment struck this section, and thus the health care reform bill as passed by the Senate does not include any provisions that address the SGR situation.

Department of Defense Appropriations Act, 2010 (P.L. 111-118)

Summary

On December 16, 2009, the House passed H.R. 3326, the FY2010 Defense Appropriations bill. One of the provisions in Section 1011 of the bill delayed the application of the update to the conversion factor until February 28, 2010.[28] Another provision in the same section reduced the amount of monies available in the Medicare Improvement Fund by $1.55 billion.[29] The Senate passed the bill on December 19, 2009,[30] and the bill was signed into law[31] that day.

Brief analysis

The bill delayed the payment reductions from taking effect for two months while maintaining fee schedule reimbursements at 2009 levels.

Increasing the Statutory Limit on the Public Debt (P.L. 111-139)

Summary

Section 7 of Title I of this bill (H.J.Res. 45, the Statutory Pay-As-You-Go Act of 2010), which was signed into law on February 12, 2010 (P.L. 111-139), provides a limited exception to the "pay-as-you-go (PAYGO)" rules for addressing the Medicare physician payment situation as a result of the SGR system (as well as additional exceptions). The maximum amount of the exception is to be the difference between estimated net outlays if 2009 Medicare fee schedule payment rates were to be in effect for the next five years (i.e., a "freeze" through December 31, 2014) and what the payments would have been had fees reverted to levels as dictated under the SGR system. Furthermore, any future legislation that reforms or replaces the SGR system would be scored for PAYGO purposes only if the modification were to cost more than the cost of the five-year freeze at 2009 levels. If legislation changing the SGR system were to be enacted that costs less than the five-year freeze through 2014, any remaining amount in the adjustment could be used to offset costs after 2014 as a result of the change, but the total adjustment could not exceed the maximum adjustment amount.

Brief Analysis

The provision exempts the equivalent of a five-year freeze of Medicare reimbursement at 2009 levels from PAYGO—an amount the CBO estimates to be $88.5 billion.[32] Congress would still have to pass legislation that would override the cuts as directed by the SGR system.

Temporary Extension Act of 2010 (P.L. 111-144)

Summary

On February 25, 2010, the House passed H.R. 4691, the Temporary Extension Act of 2010, by voice vote. This bill extended a number of expiring programs, including unemployment insurance benefits, premium assistance for COBRA benefits, and the Medicare therapy caps, in addition to forestalling the Medicare physician payment cuts. Section 5 modified the Defense Appropriations Act, 2010, by delaying the payment reduction for another month, through March 31, 2010. The CBO score for this section is $ 1.04 billion in additional outlays.[33] Although a motion to pass the bill by unanimous consent failed in the Senate that evening,[34] the bill eventually passed the Senate by a vote of 78-19[35] and was signed into law (P.L. 111-144) on March 2, 2010.

Brief Analysis

This bill delayed the payment reductions from taking effect until April 1, 2010, while maintaining fee schedule reimbursements at 2009 levels through March 31, 2010.

Tax Extenders Act of 2009 (H.R. 4213)

Summary

H.R. 4213, introduced in the House on December 7, 2009, would amend the tax code to extend certain expiring provisions and includes additional provisions. The bill passed the House by a vote of 241-181 on December 9, 2010.[36] On March 1, 2010, Senator Baucus introduced S.Amdt. 3336, which included Sec. 601, "Increase in the Medicare physician payment update." This provision would extend the 2009-level Medicare physician fee schedule reimbursements through September 30, 2010. CBO scored this provision as adding $4.71 billion in direct spending to the FY2010 budget and $1.56 billion to the FY2111 budget. On March 10, 2010, the Senate passed the amended bill, 62-36.[37]

Brief Analysis

This bill would delay the payment reductions from taking effect until October 1, 2010, while maintaining fee schedule reimbursements at 2009 levels through September 30, 2010.

Continuing Extension Act of 2010 (P.L. 111-157)

Summary

On March 17, 2010, by voice vote, the House passed H.R. 4851, as amended (striking all after the enacting clause and inserting new text). The bill includes extensions for several programs, including certain unemployment insurance provisions, premium assistance for COBRA benefits, and the Medicare therapy caps exceptions process in addition to forestalling the SGR payment reductions for another month, until May 1, 2010. The Senate amended Section 4 of the bill by lengthening the Medicare physician payment cut extension until May 31, 2010, and both houses of Congress passed the bill on April 15, 2010. The President signed the bill into law (P.L. 111-157) that day.

Brief Analysis

The bill delayed the physician payment reductions from taking effect until June 1, 2010, while maintaining fee schedule reimbursements at 2009 levels through May 31, 2010.

House Amendment to the Senate Amendment to the Tax Extenders Act of 2009 (H.R. 4213)

Summary

On May 20, 2010, the House Ways and Means Committee posted a House amendment to the Senate-passed version of H.R. 4213.[38] This amendment was further amended on May 26, 2010.[39] The resulting provision, Sec. 523, "Medicare Sustainable Growth Rate Reform," would avert the statutory payment reductions required under the SGR system from June 1, 2010, through December 31, 2011. Providers reimbursed under the Medicare fees schedule would receive a 2.2% update effective June 1, 2010, through December 31, 2010. For calendar year 2011, the update to the fee schedule would be an additional 1%. Beginning in 2012, the payment rates under the Medicare physician fee schedule would return to levels determined by the current SGR system. CBO has scored this provision as adding $22 billion to spending over the 5- and 10-year budget windows from 2010 through 2015 and 2020, respectively.[40]

The House passed the amendment to the Senate amendment to H.R. 4213 on May 28, 2010.[41]

Brief Analysis

The bill would prevent any decreases in the single update factor to the Medicare physician fee schedule through 2011 and provide updates of 2.2% for the remaining seven months of 2010 and 1% for 2011. However, the "cliff" would still return in 2012, and the magnitude of the reduction that will be required at that time by the SGR system is likely to be even greater than the 22% reduction the system currently requires.

Preservation of Access to Care for Medicare Beneficiaries and Pension Relief Act (H.R. 3962)

Summary

On June 18, 2010, more than two weeks after the May 31, 2010, expiration of the extension under the Continuing Extension Act of 2010,[42] the Senate passed an amended version of H.R. 3962 by voice vote that would avert the SGR-determined payment reduction and increase the conversion factor by 2.2% retroactive to June 1, 2010, and continuing through November 30, 2010. CBO scored this provision as adding $6.3 billion to direct spending over the 5- and 10-year budget window, with all spending occurring in fiscal years 2010 and 2011. The cost is offset (1) by imposing a three-day prohibition on hospital provision that would bar Medicare contractors from reopening or adjusting claims by hospitals during the three days preceding a patient's inpatient admission, and (2) from savings resulting from modifications that allow firms to spread out their pension fund obligations over a longer period, resulting in fewer tax-preferred contributions to pension plans and creating more taxable income for the firms.

The House passed the Senate-amended bill on June 24, 2010.[43] The President signed the bill into law (P.L. 111-192) the next day.

Brief Analysis

The act increases the Medicare physician fee schedule payments by 2.2% for six months. A substantial payment reduction (about 23%) would be required beginning December 1, 2010, and an additional reduction (about 6%) would be applied beginning January 1, 2011, in the absence of further congressional action.

End Notes

[1] 2009 Annual Report of the Boards of Trustees of the Federal Hospital Insurance And Federal Supplementary Medical Insurance Trust Funds, p. 22. http://www.cms.hhs.gov/Reports Trust Funds/downloads/tr2009.pdf.

[2] For detail on fee-for-service Medicare and other Medicare background information, see CRS Report R40425, *Medicare Primer*.

[3] Social Security Act, Sec. 1848. [42 U.S.C. 1395w–4]. In some instances, special rules apply to the calculation of Medicare fees for some services, including anesthesia, radiology, and nuclear medicine.

[4] Also called "customary, prevailing and reasonable charges," this method based physician payments on charges commonly used by physicians in a local community. The payment for a service was the lowest of (1) the physician's billed charge for the service, (2) the physician's customary charge for the service, or (3) the prevailing charge for that service in the community. For further discussion, see Physician Payment Review Commission, "Annual Report to Congress, 1997."

[5] The determination of the relative value units affects all payments under the fee schedule. Refinements in existing values and establishment of values for new services have been included in the annual fee schedule updates. This refinement and update process is based in part on recommendations made by the American Medical Association's Specialty Society Relative Value Update Committee (RUC) which receives input from approximately 100 specialty societies. The law requires a review every five years.

[6] The Balanced Budget Refinement Act of 1999 (BBRA 99, P.L. P.L. 106-113) incorporated an adjustment for the prior year into the UAF update calculation; it also moved from a fiscal year to a calendar year system.

[7] For more information on the components used to calculate the MEI and quarterly historical data, see http://www.cms.hhs.gov/MedicareProgramRatesStats/downloads/mktbskt-economic- index .pdf.

[8] See Table 6, Actual Past Medicare Economic Index Increases and Physician Updates for 1992-2009, and Estimated Values for 2010, in CMS publication, "Estimated Sustainable Growth Rate and Conversion Factor, for Medicare Payments to Physicians in 2010."

[9] CMS press release, "CMS Announces Payment, Policy Changes For Physicians Services To Medicare Beneficiaries In 2010," October 30, 2009. http://www.cms.hhs.gov/apps/media/ press/release.asp?Counter=3539&intNumPerPage=10&checkDate=&checkKey=&srchType

=1&numDays=3500&srchOpt=0&srchData=&keywordType=All&chkNewsType=1%2C+2%2C+3%2C+4%2C+5&intPage=&showAll=&pYear=&year=&desc=&cboOrder=date.

[10] U.S. Government Accountability Office (GAO), *Medicare Physician Payments: Trends in Utilization, Spending and Fees Prompt Consideration of Alternative Payment Approaches*, testimony of Bruce Steinwald before House Energy and Commerce Committee, July 25, 2006.

[11] Often referred to as the tragedy of the commons: while it may be individually rational for each herder to let livestock graze on the common field (to preserve his own), the collective consequence of many such individual decisions is that the common fields are overgrazed and all herders suffer from the degradation or depletion of the common good.

[12] See CMS Final Rule, *Medicare Program; Payment Policies Under the Physician Fee Schedule and Other Revisions to Part B for CY 2010*, to be published in the *Federal Register* on November 25, 2009.

[13] For details on Medicare Part B premiums see CRS Report R40082, *Medicare: Part B Premiums*, by Jim Hahn.

[14] P.L. 108-173, Section 953(a).

[15] U.S. Government Accountability Office, Medicare Physician Payments: Concerns about Spending Target System Prompt Interest in Considering Reforms, GAO-05-85, October 8, 2004.

[16] P.L. 109-171, Section 5104(c).

[17] Medicare Payment Advisory Commission, Assessing Alternatives to the Sustainable Growth Rate System, March 2007.

[18] MedPAC, Report to the Congress, Medicare Payment Policy, March 2008.

[19] http:// www.cbo.gov/ftpdocs/90xx/doc9055/03-14-SGR_Options.pdf.

[20] This summary and discussion includes only the proposed modifications to the Medicare physician update methodology in the CHAMP Act relevant to the ongoing discussions regarding proposed solutions.

[21] http://clerk.house.gov/cgi-bin/vote.asp?year=2007&rollnumber=787.

[22] http://www.senate.gov/legislative/LIS/roll_call_lists/roll_call_vote_cfm.cfm?congress= 111& session =1&vote= 00325.

[23] The MEI measures the weighted-average annual price change for various inputs needed to produce physicians' services. The calculation of the 2010 MEI is given in Table 33 of the final 2010 Medicare physician payment rule issued by CMS. http://www.federal register.gov/OFRUpload/OFRData/2009-26502_PI.pdf.

[24] http://clerk.house.gov/evs/2009/roll909.xml.

[25] The Senate passed the amended bill by voice vote on February 24, 2010. The House passed the Senate-amended version on February 25, 2010, by 315-97 and the bill became P.L. 111-141.

[26] CBO Cost Estimate, "H.R. 3961—Medicare Physician Payment Reform Act of 2009," November 4, 2009, http://www.cbo.gov/ftpdocs/107xx/doc10704/hr3961.pdf.

[27] http://www.senate.gov/legislative/LIS/roll_call_lists/roll_call_vote_cfm.cfm?congress= 111& session =1&vote= 00396.

[28] For roll call details, see *http://clerk.house.gov/cgi-bin/vote.asp?year=2009* & roll number=985.

[29] Section 188 of MIPPA established the Medicare Improvement Fund (MIF), available to the Secretary to make improvements under the original fee-for-service program under Parts A and B for Medicare beneficiaries.

[30] For roll call details, see http://www.senate.gov/legislative/LIS/roll_call_lists/roll_call_vote_cfm.cfm?congress=111& session=1&vote=00384.

[31] P.L. 111-118.

[32] http://www.cbo.gov/budget/factsheets/2010b/SGR-menu.pdf

[33] CBO score available at http://www.cq.com/displayfile.do?docid=3299370.

34 See the Congressional Record at http://www.congress.gov/cgi-lis/query/D?r111:2:./temp /~r111LpI3Lx.

35 http://www.senate.gov/legislative/LIS/roll_call_lists/roll_call_vote_cfm.cfm?congress=111& session =2&vote= 00032.

36 http://clerk.house.gov/cgi-bin/vote.asp?year=2009&rollnumber=943.

37 http://www.senate.gov/ legislative/LIS/roll_call_ lists/roll_call_vote_cfm.cfm? congress =111 &session =2&vote= 00048.

38 The prior version would have averted the statutory payment reductions required under the SGR system from June 1, 2010, through December 31, 2013. Providers reimbursed under the Medicare fees schedule would have received a 1.3% update effective June 1, 2010, through December 31, 2010. For calendar year 2011, the update to the fee schedule would have been an additional 1%. The provision would have reset the base year under the SGR system from 1996 to 2010, so that both target and actual expenditures for years 2012 and 2013 would have been based on 2010 expenditures. For 2012 and 2013, the annual updates would have been calculated for the two targets as defined in H.R. 3961: (1) evaluation, management, and preventive services, and (2) all other services. The target expenditures for the E&M and preventive services category would have been allowed to grow at the rate of growth of per capita GDP plus 2%, while the target expenditures for the all other category would be allowed to grow at the rate of growth of per capita GDP plus 1%. The provision would have prevented the updates for each of the service categories from being negative in those years. During this period, physicians in Accountable Care Organizations could have elected to establish ACO-specific spending targets instead of the two national spending targets. Beginning in 2014, the payment rates under the Medicare physician fee schedule would have returned to levels determined by the current SGR system. CBO scored this provision as adding $65 billion in spending. See text of the amendment at http://waysandmeans.house.gov/media/ pdf/111/HWC_711_xml.pdf.

39 http://www.rules.house.gov/111/LegText/111_hr4213_mgramnd.pdf.

40 For details, see the May 27, 2010 CBO letter to the Committee on Ways and Means, available at http://www.cbo.gov/ftpdocs/115xx/doc11531/LevinLtr_HR4213_Rules_Reported.pdf.

41 The vote was 245-117. See http://clerk.house.gov/evs/2010/roll325.xml.

42 CMS issued two instructions to its contractors regarding claims affected by the expiration. The first, on May 27, instructed contractors to hold claims for services dated June 1 and later and paid under the Medicare physician fee schedule for the first 10 business days of June (i.e., through June 14, 2010). The second, on June 18, 2010, instructed contractors to begin lifting the hold and to begin processing June 1 and later Medicare physician fee schedule claims under the law's negative update requirement on a first-in/first-out basis.

43 The vote was 417-1, with 14 members not voting. See *http://clerk.house.gov/* evs/2010/ roll393.xml.

In: Medicare Payment Policies and Issues
Editors: Alexander D. Hoffmann
ISBN: 978-1-61122-896-0

Chapter 3

MEDICARE PHYSICIAN PAYMENTS: FEES COULD BETTER REFLECT EFFICIENCIES ACHIEVED WHEN SERVICES ARE PROVIDED TOGETHER

United States Government Accountability Office

WHY GAO DID THIS STUDY

Medicare's physician fees may not always reflect efficiencies that occur when a physician performs multiple services for the same patient on the same day, and some resources required for these services do not need to be duplicated. In response to a request from Congress, GAO examined (1) the Centers for Medicare & Medicaid Services' (CMS) efforts to set appropriate fees for services furnished together and (2) additional opportunities for CMS to avoid excessive payments when services are furnished together. GAO examined relevant policies, laws, and regulations; interviewed CMS officials and others; and analyzed claims data to identify opportunities for further savings.

What GAO Recommends

GAO recommends that the Acting Administrator, CMS, ensure that physician fees reflect efficiencies occurring when services are commonly furnished together. GAO suggests that Congress consider exempting any resulting savings from federal budget neutrality so that savings accrue to Medicare. The Department of Health and Human Services concurred with GAO, stating it plans to review these services. The American Medical Association disagreed with aspects of our report, including exempting savings from budget neutrality. GAO continues to believe that Congress should consider such an exemption to help ensure appropriate payments for Medicare physician services.

What GAO Found

CMS has taken steps to ensure that physician fees recognize efficiencies that occur when certain services are commonly furnished together, that is, by the same physician to the same beneficiary on the same day, but has not targeted services with the greatest potential for savings. CMS is reviewing the efforts of a workgroup created by the American Medical Association/Specialty Society Relative Value Scale Update Committee (RUC) in 2007 to examine potential duplication in resource estimates for services furnished together. However, the RUC workgroup has not focused on services that account for the largest share of Medicare spending. For this and other reasons, its methodology to identify and review services furnished together likely will result in limited savings. The workgroup's process is also resource intensive because it depends on input and consensus from specialty societies. Independent of the RUC, CMS has implemented a multiple procedure payment reduction (MPPR) policy for certain imaging and surgical services when two or more related services are furnished together. Under an MPPR, the full fee is paid for the highest-priced service and a reduced fee is paid for each subsequent service to reflect efficiencies in overlapping portions of the practice expense component—clinical labor, supplies, and equipment. For example, a nurse's time preparing a patient for a medical procedure or technician's time setting up the required equipment is incurred only once. The MPPR produced savings of about $96 million in 2006 for imaging services. However, the scope of the policy is limited because the policy does not apply to nonsurgical and nonimaging services commonly furnished together, nor does it specifically reflect efficiencies occurring in the physician work component—the financial value of a physician's time, skill, and effort. For example, when two services are furnished together, a physician reviews a patient's medical records once, but the time for that activity is generally reflected in fees paid for both services.

CMS has additional opportunities to reduce excess physician payments that can occur when services are furnished together and Medicare's fees do not reflect the efficiencies realized. GAO's review found that expanding the MPPR to reflect practice expense efficiencies that occur when nonsurgical, nonimaging services are provided together could reduce payments for these services by an estimated one-half billion dollars annually. GAO's review also indicated that expanding the existing MPPR policy to reflect efficiencies in the physician work component of certain imaging services could reduce these payments by an estimated additional $175 million annually. Under the budget neutrality requirement, by law, savings from reductions in fees are redistributed by increasing fees for all other services. Thus, these potential savings would accrue as savings to Medicare only if Congress exempted them from the budget neutrality requirement, as was done in the Deficit Reduction Act of 2005 for savings from the changes to certain imaging services fees.

ABBREVIATIONS

AMA	American Medical Association
CMS	Centers for Medicare & Medicaid Services
CPT®	Current Procedural Terminology
CT	computed tomography
DRA	Deficit Reduction Act of 2005
HHS	Department of Health and Human Services
MedPAC	Medicare Payment Advisory Commission
MPPR	multiple procedure payment reduction
RBRVS	Resource-Based Relative Value Scale
RUC	AMA/Specialty Society Relative Value Scale Update Committee
RVU	relative value unit

July 31, 2009

The Honorable Frank Pallone
Chairman
The Honorable Nathan Deal
Ranking Member
Subcommittee on Health
Committee on Energy and Commerce
House of Representatives

The Honorable Pete Stark
Chairman
Subcommittee on Health
Committee on Ways and Means
House of Representatives

The Honorable Dave Camp
Ranking Member
Committee on Ways and Means
House of Representatives

Spending on Medicare Part B physician services grew at an average annual rate of 6 percent from 1997 through 2008, more than twice the growth rate in the national economy over this period.[1] This rapid spending growth underscores the importance of ensuring that payments under Medicare's physician fee schedule, which includes fees for each of over 7,000 services, such as office visits, surgical procedures, and tests, are appropriate and encourage efficient use of resources.

Physician fee schedule payments may be excessive for some services because efficiencies that occur when two or more services are furnished together are not reflected in the fee schedule, and thus Medicare essentially pays twice for the portions of these services that overlap. In setting payments for services under the fee schedule, the Centers for Medicare & Medicaid Services (CMS)—the federal agency that administers the Medicare program—estimates resources required to provide three separate components of each service: the physician work component (which reflects the physician's time, skill, and effort); the practice expense component (which reflects operating expenses, such as rent, utilities, and the salaries of nurses, technicians, and administrative staff); and the malpractice component (which reflects the costs of obtaining professional liability insurance).[2] Each service is generally considered to be discrete and stand-alone. But when two or more services are furnished by the same physician to the same beneficiary on the same day, efficiencies may occur because some portions of the physician work component, the practice expense component, or both overlap and are incurred only once. For example, certain physician work activities—such as reviewing the patient's medical history or dictating a report for the medical record and following up with the referring physician after a medical procedure—occur only once. Similarly, certain practice expenses—such as a nurse's time spent in obtaining the patient's consent and preparing the patient for the procedure, or a technician's time in setting up the required equipment—are incurred only once. However, payment for these overlapping portions is generally included in each fee, resulting in excessive payments by Medicare.[3]

You asked us to explore options to ensure that the physician fee schedule appropriately reflects efficiencies occurring across all types of services that are commonly furnished together. This report examines (1) CMS's current efforts to ensure that Medicare physician fees reflect efficiencies in services commonly furnished together and (2) additional opportunities for CMS to avoid excessive payments for Medicare physician services commonly furnished together.

To determine how CMS ensures that Medicare physician fees reflect efficiencies for services commonly furnished together, we reviewed CMS's relevant payment policies and applicable laws and regulations. We interviewed officials from several organizations to discuss other instances where the physician fee schedule could better reflect efficiencies for these services. These organizations included CMS, the Medicare Payment Advisory Commission (MedPAC), and 7 of the 15 Medicare contractors that process and pay Part B claims.[4] We also met with representatives from the American Medical Association (AMA) and AMA-sponsored physician panels that assist CMS in developing estimates of resources required to deliver physician fee schedule services to discuss their initiatives to refine resource estimates for services commonly furnished together.

To determine additional opportunities for CMS to avoid excessive payments for services that are commonly furnished together, we conducted a systematic review of all pairs of services furnished by the same physician to the same beneficiary on the same day from 2006 Medicare claims data.[5] We excluded pairs subject to an existing Medicare billing or payment policy that reflected efficiencies when these services were furnished together. From the remaining service pairs, we selected the 350 that accounted for the highest share of Medicare spending and met with Medicare contractor Medical Directors and their staffs in five different states to determine whether efficiencies occurred in any of these service pairs. We also consulted with other experts from three medical specialty societies and reviewed AMA resource estimates of physician work and practice expenses.[6] On the basis of these discussions and analyses, we estimated resulting savings to the Medicare program if fees were adjusted to reflect efficiencies occurring in the service pairs identified by the contractors. Our estimate of savings is based upon the premise that providers do not change their practice patterns (for example, by scheduling services on different days) in response to these fee adjustments. Appendix I provides more detailed information on our methodology to estimate the potential for further savings from service pairs commonly furnished together.

We examined the reliability of the claims data used in this report by performing appropriate electronic checks, including those for obvious errors, such as missing values and values outside of expected ranges. We also interviewed officials who were knowledgeable about the data, including CMS and Medicare contractor officials. We determined that the claims data we used were sufficiently reliable for purposes of our analysis because they are used by the Medicare program as a record of payments to health care providers. As such, they are subject to routine CMS scrutiny.

We conducted our work from May 2008 through July 2009 in accordance with generally accepted government auditing standards. Those standards require that we plan and perform the audit to obtain sufficient, appropriate evidence to provide a reasonable basis for our findings and conclusions based on our audit objectives. We believe that the evidence obtained provides a reasonable basis for our findings and conclusions based on our audit objectives.

BACKGROUND

Medicare's physician fee schedule includes payments for over 7,000 services, such as office visits, surgical procedures, and tests.[7] Most services are defined as discrete and stand-alone in that they may be furnished independently of other services, but a small number of services are defined as supplemental because they are commonly furnished along with other primary services.

Process for Defining Medicare Fee Schedule Services

Services under the Medicare fee schedule are described and defined by the AMA's Current Procedural Terminology (CPT) Editorial Panel, and each service is assigned a five-digit identifier, or code. The CPT Editorial Panel revises and modifies CPT codes based largely on suggestions from specialty societies and the CPT Editorial Panel's Advisory Committee.[8] Code revisions require research from both CPT staff and specialty society members who assist the CPT Editorial Panel in its work. According to AMA officials, the CPT process generally takes about 14 months from the time potential codes are first identified by specialty societies to the final revision or development of a new code.

Process for Developing and Updating Resource Estimates Used to Set Fees

CMS relies on the AMA/Specialty Society Relative Value Scale Update Committee (RUC)—an expert panel that includes members from national physician specialty societies—to develop and update on an ongoing basis the resource estimates upon which fees are based.[9] Specialty societies identify services for review, gather data on resource use, and make proposals to the RUC on resource estimates for services. Physician work estimates are developed using vignettes of each service furnished to a typical patient, where the specific physician activities are described for three phases—before, during, and after the service.[10] Practice expense estimates considered direct—clinical labor (that is, the nurse's or technician's time), equipment, and supplies—are developed similarly for each of these phases.[11,12] (App. II provides an example of a vignette and practice expense estimates for one service.) The RUC evaluates proposals submitted by the specialty societies and makes recommendations for final consideration by CMS. The RUC meets three times a year, and, on average, reviews approximately 300 codes annually. The RUC also assists CMS in the Five-Year Review process—a review of fees for all services that the agency is required by law to conduct at least every 5 years to account for changes in medical practice.[13]

While CMS may reject or modify the RUC's recommendations, from 1993 through 2009, the agency accepted over 90 percent of the recommendations pertaining to 3,600 new and revised CPT codes. CMS may at times also make changes to fees for services independent of RUC recommendations.

Initiatives to Account for Efficiencies in Multiple Services

Efficiencies in multiple services that are furnished together may be factored into fees primarily in two ways. First, the RUC and specialty societies generally attempt to consider whether other services are typically furnished along with the service they are reviewing to avoid duplication of the resources associated with physician work and practice expenses that may be incurred only once. For example, certain activities included in the practice expense component, such as preparing the patient before a procedure and cleaning the room after the procedure, are performed only once when two services are furnished together. However, the RUC has not reviewed every service; therefore, estimates are outdated for a large portion of services and may no longer reflect current technology and medical practice. For example, resource estimates for certain image-guided surgeries were developed when a surgeon performed the surgery and a radiologist performed the related imaging, whereas in current medical practice, a single physician tends to do both tasks. Further, for supplemental services, the RUC ensures that the physician work and practice expense resources required before and after the service are not duplicated.

Second, CMS has, independent of the RUC and specialty societies, implemented its own policies to recognize efficiencies occurring in certain services. CMS has a long-standing policy called a multiple procedure payment reduction (MPPR) to avoid duplicate payments for portions of practice expenses that are incurred only once when two or more surgical services are furnished together by the same physician during the same operating session.[14] CMS expanded the MPPR to include certain diagnostic imaging services in 2006.[15] Under the MPPR policy, the full fee is paid for the more expensive service, but a reduction is applied to the fees for each subsequent service. Generally, a 50 percent reduction is applied to fees for surgical services performed during the same operating session and a 25 percent reduction is applied to fees for certain imaging services that are furnished together.[16]

Budget Neutrality

By law, updates to fees are required to be budget neutral—that is, they cannot cause Medicare's aggregate payments to physicians to increase or decrease by more than $20 million.[17] As a result, any "savings" realized from reducing the fees for particular services do not accrue to the Medicare program but are redistributed across all services, resulting in a slight increase to the fees for all other services. In some instances, Congress has overridden budget neutrality to ensure that payment changes result in savings to Medicare. For example, through the Deficit Reduction Act of 2005 (DRA), Congress mandated that savings resulting from the MPPR for certain imaging services that were furnished together be exempted from budget neutrality.[18] As a result, annual savings of approximately $96 million were not redistributed across all services, but accrued as savings to the Medicare program in 2006.

CMS Has Recognized Efficiencies in Some Services, but Has Not Focused on High-Spending Services

CMS has taken steps to recognize efficiencies for services commonly furnished together through the use of the RUC process and the MPPR, but has not targeted services with the greatest potential for savings, and the RUC process depends on specialty societies. The MPPR is limited in scope because it does not apply to a broad range of services, nor does it capture efficiencies occurring in the physician work component.

RUC Workgroup Examines Efficiencies in Services Commonly Furnished Together, but Does Not Target Services with Greatest Potential for Savings

CMS stated that it is reviewing the efforts of a workgroup recently created by the RUC to identify efficiencies in services that are commonly furnished together. In March 2006 MedPAC criticized the RUC for recommending more increases than decreases in resource estimates, largely because the RUC had focused on services that specialty societies believed were undervalued. In response, the RUC established the Five-Year Review Identification

Workgroup in October 2006 to identify potentially misvalued services. The workgroup used several criteria to identify these services, one of which was to examine services commonly furnished together to determine if such services should be bundled to reduce duplication in the physician work component. The workgroup requested data from CMS on services commonly furnished together in 2007. CMS forwarded a list of over 2,200 service pairs that were furnished together more than 50 percent of the time, but did not tell the workgroup how to prioritize its review of the services. Instead, the workgroup developed its own methodology, targeting service pairs that were almost exclusively furnished together.

While the methodology represents a reasonable first step to identify potentially misvalued services, and the workgroup has expended considerable effort and resources in implementing it, the methodology will likely result in limited savings to Medicare. This is because the group did not systematically focus on services that accounted for a large share of Medicare spending, nor did it exclude supplemental services with limited potential for savings.

The workgroup focused on service pairs in which the two services were performed together at least 90 percent of the time. The workgroup classified service pairs into two types: type A, in which both services in the pair were performed together at least 90 percent of the time, and type B, in which one service was performed with another service at least 90 percent of the time in a unidirectional relationship (that is, when the first service was performed, the second service was also performed at least 90 percent of the time, but when the second service was performed, the first service was not performed at least 90 percent of the time). The workgroup identified 22 type A and 31 type B service pairs where possible duplication was occurring in physician work.[19]

However, these service pairs would likely result in limited savings. First, 19 of the 22 type A pairs and 20 of the 31 type B pairs included supplemental services for which further reductions in fees would likely be small. For example, in performing a three-dimensional heart wall imaging study (also known as a myocardial perfusion imaging study), physicians may take additional measurements of blood flow or heart wall function. These additional services are supplemental to the primary service and are therefore already priced to exclude overlap in practice expenses incurred before and after the service. Second, spending for the lower-priced service in the remaining pairs was minimal: $27 million for the remaining 3 type A services and $117 million for the remaining 11 type B services. Thus, potential savings from combining the remaining service pairs would likely be no more than half these respective amounts, assuming a 50 percent discount was applied to the lower-priced service—a generous assumption, since that is the maximum discount that CMS has applied to services under the MPPR.

Another limitation of the workgroup's review of services commonly furnished together is that its process is resource intensive. This element is inherent in a process based on input and consensus from specialty societies. The workgroup follows the RUC's process in that it solicits proposals from specialty societies for potential revisions to the service pairs. The proposals must then be approved by the CPT Editorial Panel, the RUC, and CMS (see figure 1).

To date, the workgroup has identified only a limited number of misvalued services commonly furnished together. Since the review of service pairs that was started in 2007, the workgroup has identified three misvalued services; at the workgroup's recommendation, these (echocardiography) services were combined into a single code in 2009. The earliest any additional changes might be implemented for the type A and B service pairs first identified in 2007 would be 2010.[20]

Finally, the workgroup is required to undertake other tasks, including reviewing services because of technological changes or because of high growth, utilization, or intensity.[21] These reviews also require involvement from the specialty societies, in addition to their efforts to revise estimates of physician work and practice expenses an ongoing basis as well as for the Five-Year Reviews. Despite the demands of these tasks, the RUC has stated that CMS should continue to rely on the workgroup to identify opportunities for efficiencies, rather than implement an MPPR, which it perceives to be an imprecise tool for reducing duplicate payments for portions of services furnished only once.

CMS's MPPR Policy Reflects Efficiencies but Is Limited in Scope

CMS's MPPR policy reflects efficiencies for certain imaging and surgical procedures commonly furnished together, but it is limited in scope. CMS estimated that its use of the MPPR for certain imaging procedures produced savings of about $96 million in 2006.[22,23] In this instance, Congress exempted these savings from the budget neutrality provision; as a result, the $96 million was not redirected to other services but accrued as savings to the Medicare program.

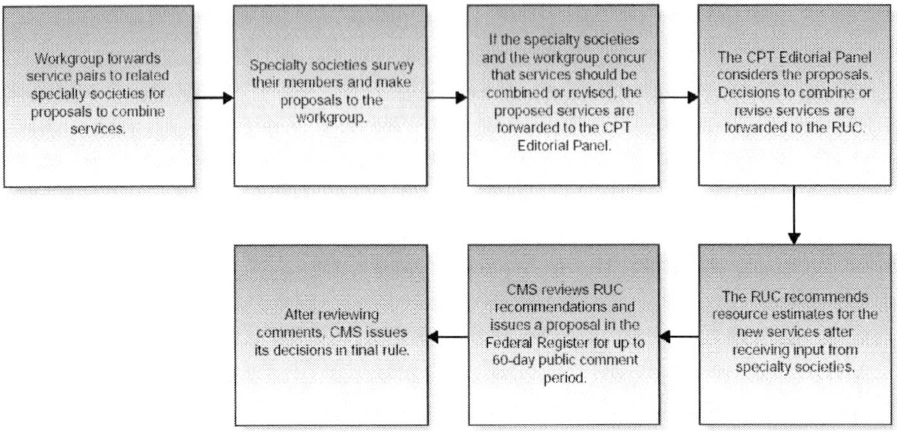

Source: GAO analysis.

Figure 1. Overview of Workgroup Process to Identify Misvalued Services Furnished by the Same Physician to the Same Beneficiary on the Same Day

In principle, an MPPR can be implemented quickly to reflect efficiencies for services performed together. In developing the list of services to be selected for an MPPR, CMS does not formally solicit opinion from specialty societies or others until the MPPR is published as a proposed rule. For example, in developing the imaging MPPR, CMS—acting independently of the RUC and specialty societies, on MedPAC's recommendation—identified imaging services that were commonly furnished together and determined an appropriate discount to account for efficiencies occurring in the practice expense component.[24] CMS then published these decisions in its August 2005 proposed rule for specialty society and public comment and finalized its decisions in November 2005 after evaluating and responding to stakeholder comments. These changes went into effect on January 1, 2006.

The MPPR as currently used by CMS does have limitations. First, the MPPR does not apply to nonsurgical and nonimaging services that are commonly furnished together. When CMS developed the MPPR for surgical services in 1996, it acknowledged that efficiencies likely also occur for nonsurgical services. However, other than the imaging MPPR, CMS has not implemented an MPPR policy for nonsurgical services.[25] Contractors we interviewed identified many opportunities to expand the MPPR policy to areas where services are commonly furnished together. For example, they stated that similar efficiencies occur when certain types of tests—such as nerve conduction studies or pulmonary function, vision, and hearing tests—are performed together. However, as of July 2009, CMS had not published proposals to systematically review services commonly furnished together by focusing on the most expensive services with the greatest potential for savings to Medicare.

Second, the MPPR only reflects efficiencies occurring in practice expenses, not in the physician work component, where certain physician activities may occur only once.[26] For example, a physician's review of a patient's medical history and prior imaging or other test results before the service, and dictation of the final report for the medical record, occur only once. Under the current payment methodology, the time spent on these activities is included in each service because the services are assumed to be furnished separately. Several organizations we interviewed stated that an MPPR for the physician work component was warranted to avoid duplicate payments to physicians for activities that they perform only once. In its 2006 report, MedPAC similarly recommended that CMS examine efficiencies that might be occurring in the physician work component but are not reflected in the fee schedule.[27] However, CMS has not conducted such a review.

CMS's MPPR Policy Could be Applied to other Services Commonly Furnished Together and Expanded to Reflect Efficiencies in Physician Work

Our review of Medicare claims data indicated the potential for reducing excessive physician payments by implementing an MPPR to reflect efficiencies generally occurring in the practice expense component of certain nonsurgical and nonimaging service pairs commonly furnished together. In addition, our analysis of certain imaging services indicated potential for further reducing excessive payments by implementing an MPPR to reflect efficiencies in the physician work component when these services are performed together.

Potential Exists for Reducing at Least One-Half Billion Dollars in Excessive Payments Annually through an MPPR to Reflect Efficiencies in the Practice Expense Component

Our systematic review of a sample of the most costly service pairs showed potential for annual savings of over one-half billion dollars with implementation of an MPPR to reflect efficiencies in the practice expense component. Contractor Medical Directors we met with determined that an MPPR was appropriate for 149 (over 40 percent) of the 350 most costly service pairs we reviewed with them. The contractor Medical Directors recommended these MPPRs to reflect efficiencies occurring in practice expenses for services that were furnished only once. The 149 service pairs included interventional radiology procedures, physical therapy services, and various tests, such as additional imaging, pulmonary function, vision, hearing, and pathology.[28] For example, a cardiovascular stress test is commonly furnished with a three-dimensional heart imaging test. However, the Medical Directors cautioned that CMS would need to carefully monitor utilization of these services to ensure that physicians did not change their behavior by scheduling services on different days to avoid reduced fees for those subject to an MPPR.

Potential Exists for Reducing about $175 Million Annually through Expanding the Current MPPR for Imaging Services to Reflect Efficiencies in the Physician Work Component

Our analysis of 118 imaging service pairs suggests that efficiencies in physician work occur when services are furnished together, and an MPPR policy that reflected these efficiencies could save Medicare over $175 million annually.[29] We sought the advice of contractor Medical Directors and other experts, who agreed that efficiencies occur in physician work when two or more services are furnished together and that an MPPR would be appropriate to account for these efficiencies. Our savings estimate is based on reducing fees for the lower-priced service in each service pair to reflect efficiencies in physician time spent on activities performed before and after the service that are already included in the higher-priced service. For example, the service pair that accounted for the largest share of spending across all imaging service pairs was the physician's interpretation of two computed tomography (CT) scans: CT of the abdomen with dye and CT of the pelvis with dye.[30] Of a total of 18 minutes allotted for interpretation of the second (lower-priced) service, 8 minutes were allotted for activities such as reviewing the patient's prior medical history before the service and reviewing the final report and following up with the referring physician after the service. Since time spent on these activities was already included in the first (higher-priced) service, we discounted the fee for the lower-priced service by 44 percent (that is, 8 minutes ÷ 18 minutes).[31] While the results of our analysis cannot be generalized to all service pairs, the concept of applying an MPPR for the physician work component could be applied to other services.

Our analysis focused on efficiencies in activities performed before and after each service, but there are also likely efficiencies occurring during, or within, the intraservice phase. For example, a practicing radiologist we interviewed stated that when two CT scans of contiguous body areas (e.g., the abdomen and pelvis) are taken at the same time, the total number of actual CT images reviewed is lower than if each scan were performed separately. This is because an abdominal CT generally includes margins of the pelvis and vice versa, and the images of these overlapping margins are examined only once by the radiologist. Other efficiencies relating to technology advances, such as digital storage and retrieval of imaging, may also be realized during the intraservice phase.

CONCLUSIONS

The RUC and specialty societies may be limited in their ability to help CMS quickly identify opportunities for further savings from efficiencies occurring when services are commonly furnished together. The RUC's methodology for identifying additional services is not focused on finding savings for the Medicare program. Moreover, the RUC workgroup's dependence on specialty societies limits its ability to make progress. CMS, on the other hand, has the tools in place to readily expand its MPPR policy to reflect efficiencies occurring in the practice expense and physician work components of services that are commonly furnished together. However, as of July 2009, the agency did not appear to have conducted a systematic review of claims data to identify opportunities with the greatest potential for further savings. Further, unless specifically exempted by Congress (as was done in the DRA for fee changes for certain imaging services), savings would be redistributed to other services in accordance with the budget neutrality provision, and the Medicare program would not realize savings.

Recommendation for Executive Action

The Acting Administrator of CMS should take further steps to ensure that fees for services paid under Medicare's physician fee schedule reflect efficiencies that occur when services are performed by the same physician to the same beneficiary on the same day. These efforts could include

- systematically reviewing services commonly furnished together and implementing an MPPR to capture efficiencies in both physician work and practice expenses, where appropriate, for these services;
- focusing on service pairs that have the most impact on Medicare spending; and
- monitoring the provision of services affected by any new policies it implements to ensure that physicians do not change their behavior in response to these policies.

Matter for Congressional Consideration

To ensure that savings are realized from the implementation of an MPPR or other policies that reflect efficiencies occurring when services are furnished together, Congress should consider exempting these savings from budget neutrality.

Agency and Professional Association Comments and Our Evaluation

We obtained written comments on a draft of this report from the Department of Health and Human Services (HHS), which are reprinted in appendix III. We obtained oral comments from representatives of the AMA.

HHS Comments

HHS concurred with our recommendation and stated that CMS plans to perform an analysis of nonsurgical codes that are furnished together between 60 and 70 percent of the time to determine whether efficiencies occur in the physician work and practice expense component of these services. HHS stated that it would implement policies to reflect these efficiencies, as appropriate, and agreed that CMS should focus on service pairs that have the most impact on Medicare spending. HHS also agreed on the need to monitor physician utilization of services if the MPPR is expanded. HHS suggested that we include in an appendix to the report the specific service pairs that we identified.

We did not include such an appendix because our report focuses on illustrating the value of CMS's taking a more systematic approach, rather than focusing on specific service pairs, to ensure that the fee schedule reflects efficiencies when services are provided together. However, we will work with CMS officials and share information to aid in the agency's efforts.

AMA Comments

AMA representatives expressed three broad concerns about the draft report. First, they disagreed with our assessment of the RUC workgroup's efforts to ensure that services are appropriately coded and valued. Second, they stated that a broad application of the MPPR to account for efficiencies in practice expenses and physician work was not appropriate. Third, they opposed our matter for congressional consideration that suggests that any savings from implementing the report's recommendations be exempted from budget neutrality requirements.

RUC Workgroup's Efforts

AMA representatives disagreed with the report draft's characterization of the efficacy of the RUC workgroup, noting that the RUC workgroup's efforts have been aggressive, timely, and efficient. They also stated that the specialty societies had developed proposals to combine the type A and B service pairs that would result in significant savings should CMS implement them in 2010 or 2011. As an example, they projected that the proposals to combine 14 myocardial perfusion services of the workgroup's 53 type A and type B service pairs would result in annual savings of about $40 million from efficiencies occurring in the physician work component. In addition, they said that while they did not have an estimate, they believed that savings for the practice expense component would also likely be significant. Finally, representatives stated that in its review of potentially misvalued services, the workgroup may have already identified and made recommendations on some of the unique codes or pairs included in our list of 149 code pairs.

We acknowledge in the draft the time and effort the workgroup has expended in identifying potentially misvalued services. However, based on our review of the workgroup's processes and progress to date, we continue to believe that these processes are resource intensive and will likely limit CMS's ability to quickly identify opportunities for savings from those service pairs that account for a high share of Medicare spending. In addition, as stated in the draft, the workgroup has not prioritized its review to systematically focus on services with the greatest potential savings for Medicare. While it is possible that some of the type A and type B service pairs the workgroup identified may be relatively costly, its methodology does not systematically focus on such services. We believe our assessment of the workgroup's progress remains accurate—as of 2009 the workgroup had identified only three misvalued services that were combined. Finally, from our list of 149 code pairs (which included 116 unique codes), the workgroup had identified only one code pair and 21 unique codes in its review of potentially misvalued codes.

Broader Application of MPPR

AMA representatives stated that a "blanket reduction" of 25 percent for the 149 code pairs based on duplication in time spent on certain preservice and postservice tasks was not appropriate. They contended that for an average service, the intensity of time spent on tasks in the preservice and postservice phases is less than the intensity of time spent on intraservice tasks. AMA representatives added that in some instances a 25 percent reduction may be too high, whereas in other instances it might be more appropriate. They said that for some of the newer codes, the RUC had already taken any potential efficiencies into account, but for some of the old codes, which have not been revalued by the RUC, the 25 percent discount may be more reasonable. The AMA representatives also stated that the RUC workgroup's efforts result in a more accurate and credible system of coding and valuation of services and thus is more effective than the application of "arbitrary policies" such as an MPPR.

In the draft report, we acknowledge the limitations of our approach and state that the results of our analysis cannot be generalized to all service pairs. Our draft also states that the discount of 25 percent we applied to the 149 code pairs is consistent with the imaging MPPR that reflects efficiencies in the practice expense component. We do not recommend that CMS adopt our specific methodology; rather we present it as an illustration of potential efficiencies occurring in the physician work component that can be uncovered through a systematic review of service pairs. However, we continue to believe that CMS should undertake a systematic review of services and, where appropriate, expand the MPPR to ensure that physician fee schedule payments reflect efficiencies when services are performed by the same physician to the same beneficiary on the same day.

Exempting Savings from Budget Neutrality Requirement

AMA representatives disagreed with the draft's statement that spending on physician services has recently grown at an average annual rate of 6 percent, and opposed our suggestion that Congress consider exempting any savings from implementation of the report's recommendations from federal budget neutrality requirements. AMA representatives told us that the growth rate of per beneficiary spending on Part B physician services has slowed to an annual rate of 3 percent in 2006 and 2007. Regarding our suggestion that Congress consider exempting any savings from budget neutrality, AMA representatives expressed concern that the exemption would have an adverse effect on primary care services that could benefit from the redistribution of savings and stated that savings would be spent on other programs.

We agree that the annual rate of growth in per beneficiary spending on physician services slowed somewhat in 2006 and 2007, but even taking this into account, annual spending from 1997 to 2008 grew an average of 6 percent. We recommend that Congress consider exempting potential savings from budget neutrality to help ensure the fiscal health of the Medicare program. As we noted in the draft, there is recent precedent for exempting savings from budget neutrality. We agree that primary care services are important, but Congress has other mechanisms for altering payment for these services.

AMA representatives also provided technical comments, which we incorporated as appropriate.

APPENDIX I: ESTIMATING POTENTIAL FOR FURTHER SAVINGS FROM EFFICIENCIES IN MULTIPLE SERVICE

In this appendix, we describe the processes we used to determine opportunities for the Centers for Medicare & Medicaid Services (CMS) to avoid excessive payments for services commonly furnished together.

Estimating Potential for Further Savings from Efficiencies in the Practice Expense Component of Multiple Services through Systematic Review of Medicare Claims Data

To determine additional opportunities for CMS to avoid excessive payments for services that are commonly furnished together, we conducted a systematic review of Medicare claims data using the 2006 Medicare Physician/Supplier Part B 5 Percent Standard Analytic File.[32] To conduct this review, we selected physician services that were paid under the resource-based payment methodology.[33] We generated a list of all service pairs that were furnished by the same physician to the same beneficiary on the same day and made the following exclusions:

- service pairs with low utilization—those that were billed fewer than 5,000 times annually;
- service pairs containing only the professional portion of a service;[34]
- service pairs that were already subject to payment policies that reduced payments for one of the services in the pair;[35]
- service pairs containing supplemental services, which are priced to exclude duplication of physician work and practice expenses that are already included in the primary service;[36] and
- service pairs containing duplicate services.

The remaining list of service pairs was our universe of pairs that represented opportunities for savings from efficiencies that resulted when the two services were furnished together.[37] To target our review to the service pairs that accounted for a large share of Medicare spending, we ranked the service pairs based on spending for the lesser-priced service (since the multiple procedure payment reduction (MPPR) and other policies usually apply to that service) and selected the 350 costliest service pairs based on total spending. We met with contractor Medical Directors and their staffs in five different states to determine if there were efficiencies taking place in the practice expense component when these service pairs were furnished together. To ensure consistency of review across the five contractors, we developed a standard set of questions that each contractor followed in evaluating the service pairs. We asked contractors to examine service descriptions and definitions, as well as coding instructions from the Current Procedural Terminology (CPT) manual and from CMS, and use their clinical judgment and knowledge to assess whether there were efficiencies occurring because certain practice expenses were incurred only once before and after each service in the service pairs. We also asked contractors to determine the payment policy that best captured these efficiencies. For example, contractors determined whether the services in each pair should be combined into a single code, there should be no payment for one service in the service pair because it was inherently included in the other, or an MPPR should be applied. If an MPPR should be applied, contractors determined the approximate discount that was most appropriate. Since all five contractors determined that an MPPR was the most appropriate payment policy to reflect efficiencies in all 149 of the 350 service pairs they identified as having potential, we estimated total savings to the Medicare program by applying the appropriate discount to spending for the lower-priced service in each pair.

Our estimate of savings is conservative for several reasons. First, we excluded services that were billed multiple times on the same day by the same physician, since our focus was on potential savings when two unique services were furnished together. To the extent that there is overlap of physician work and practice expenses in the preservice and postservice phases of these duplicate services, an MPPR should be applied to account for this overlap. Second, we generally applied a discount of 25 percent or less to the service pairs to mirror CMS's discount on imaging service pairs, although, in certain instances, a higher discount was warranted based on the extent of duplication in practice expenses.

Estimating Potential Savings from an MPPR to Reflect Efficiencies in Physician Work Component

To estimate potential savings from applying an MPPR to account for duplication of physician work activities occurring before and after each service in the service pairs, we first examined the American Medical Association

(AMA) database—the Resource-Based Relative Value System (RBRVS) Data Manager—to determine if data on these activities were available for all service pairs. The RBRVS Data Manager contains vignettes describing the physician's work for a specific procedure for a typical patient in three phases: preservice, intraservice, and postservice.[38] The AMA/Specialty Society Relative Value Scale Update Committee (RUC) bases its estimates of physician work and practice expenses on these vignettes. Because we found that vignettes were missing for a large proportion of services, we used physician time—the amount of time it takes a physician to perform a service—as a proxy for physician work, and discounted the fee for the lesser-priced service in each service pair for the extent of overlap in physician time spent on the preservice and postservice phases across the two services.[39] Using the physician time file on the CMS Web site, we calculated this discount as the sum of time spent on the preservice and postservice phases of the lesser-priced service divided by total time for that service.[40] We limited our analysis to the imaging service pairs that we had identified from our review of Medicare claims data because we wanted to examine a homogenous group of services where the activities included in the pre- and postservice phases were generally the same across different imaging services, and therefore the time spent on pre- and postservice phases was also likely to be relatively uniform across this group of services. We applied the discount to the professional fee of imaging services, since the professional fee captures the physician's work in interpreting the imaging service. We discussed our approach with several experts in the Medicare physician payment system. These included an experienced contractor Medical Director; a Medicare Payment Advisory Commission (MedPAC) official who is an expert in Medicare physician payment policy; and a practicing radiologist and leading expert in the field who has written extensively on Medicare payment policy and reimbursement issues. They concurred that our methodology was a reasonable approach to estimating potential savings from an MPPR for physician work.

APPENDIX II: EXAMPLES OF VIGNETTE AND PRACTICE EXPENSE ESTIMATE

This appendix contains examples of a vignette and a practice expense estimate. The vignette (figure 2) is used by specialty societies to develop estimates of physician work resources for a service. The practice expense estimate (figure 3) describes the nonphysician clinical labor, supplies, and equipment resources required for each service.

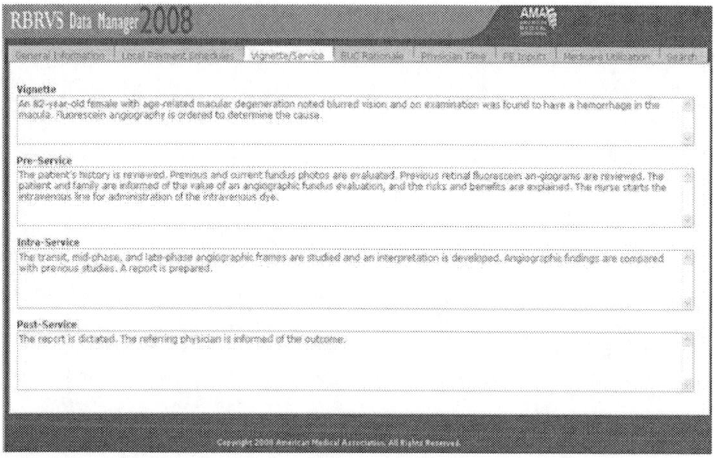

Source: 2008 American Medical Association.

Figure 2. Example of AMA Vignette for CPT Code 92235, Eye Exam with Photos

AMA/Specialty Society RVS Update Committee Recommendations		
LOCATION: In-office	CMS STAFF TYPE, MEDICAL SUPPLY, OR EQUIPMENT CODE	CPT code: 92235 Code Descriptor: Eye Exam with Photos
TOTAL CLINICAL LABOR TIME		67
SERVICE PERIOD		
Start: When patient enters office for surgery/procedure		
Pre-service:		
Review charts	Certified Retinal Angiographer	2
Greet patient and provide gowning	Certified Retinal Angiographer	2
Obtain vital signs		
Provide pre-service education/obtain consent	Certified Retinal Angiographer	5
Prepare room, equipment, supplies		
Prepare and position patient/monitor patient/set up IV	RN/Other	10
Sedate/apply anesthesia		
Intra-service		
Assist physician in performing procedure	Certified Retinal Angiographer	40
Post-service		
Monitor patient following service/check tubes, monitor drains	RN/Other	5
Clean room/equipment by physician staff		
Complete diagnostic forms, lab and X-ray requisitions		
Review/read X-ray, lab and pathology reports		
Label and file photos/slides with patient chart	Certified Retinal Angiographer	3
Other clinical activity (please specify)		
End: Patient leaves office		
MEDICAL SUPPLIES		
Pack, ophthalmology visit (w-dilation)	SA082	1
Applicator, cotton-tipped, non-sterile 6in	SG008	2
IV infusion set	SC018	1
18 gauge filter needle	SC027	1
Needle, butterfly 20 to 25 gauge	SC030	1
Syringe 5-6 ml	SC057	1
Band aid 3/4"x3"	SG021	2
Fluorescein inj (5ml uou)	SH033	1
Povidone soln, (Betadine)	SJ041	10
Film, Tri-x 35mm BW (per exposure)	SK030	24
Paper, photo printing (8.5 x 11)	SK058	2
Photographic stop bath	SK065	8
EQUIPMENT		
Electric table	EF030	1
Exam Lane	EL005	1
Topcon Retinal Camera, incl. monitor, printer, etc. ($78,000)	ED008	1

Source: American Medical Association.

Figure 3. Example of AMA Practice Expense Estimates for CPT Code 92235, Eye Exam with Photos

APPENDIX III: COMMENTS FROM THE DEPARTMENT OF HEALTH AND HUMAN SERVICES

DEPARTMENT OF HEALTH & HUMAN SERVICES | OFFICE OF THE SECRETARY

Assistant Secretary for Legislation
Washington, DC 20201

JUL 6 2009

James Cosgrove
Director, Health Care
U.S. Government Accountability Office
441 G Street N.W.
Washington, DC 20548

Dear Mr. Cosgrove:

Enclosed are comments on the U.S. Government Accountability Office's (GAO) report entitled: "MEDICARE PHYSICIAN PAYMENTS: Fees Could Better Reflect Efficiencies Achieved When Services Are Provided Together" (GAO-09-647).

The Department appreciates the opportunity to review this report before its publication.

Sincerely,

Barbara Pisaro Clark
Acting Assistant Secretary for Legislation

Attachment

DEPARTMENT OF HEALTH & HUMAN SERVICES

Centers for Medicare & Medicaid Services

200 Independence Avenue SW
Washington, DC 20201

DATE: JUL 0 2 2009

TO: Barbara Pisaro Clark
Assistant Secretary for Legislation

FROM: Charlene Frizzera
Acting Administrator

SUBJECT: Government Accountability Office's Report: "MEDICARE PHYSICIAN PAYMENTS: Fees Could Better Reflect Efficiencies Achieved When Services Are Provided Together" (GAO-09-647)

Thank you for the opportunity to review and comment on the Government Accountability Office's (GAO) draft report entitled "MEDICARE PHYSICIAN PAYMENTS: Fees Could Better Reflect Efficiencies Achieved When Services Are Provided Together."

Medicare has a longstanding policy of reducing payment for multiple surgical procedures performed on the same patient, by the same physician, on the same day. The multiple procedure payment reduction (MPPR) for surgery is largely based on the efficiencies recognized in practice expenses for pre and post-surgical services.

In 1995, the MPPR was extended to six nuclear medicine diagnostic procedures performed on the same patient on the same day. For surgical and nuclear medicine diagnostic procedures, payment is made in full for the highest priced procedure, and at 50 percent for the second procedure.

In 2006, the MPPR was extended to certain diagnostic imaging procedures performed on contiguous areas of the body in the same session. In such cases, most clinical labor activities and most supplies are not performed or furnished twice. The payment reduction applies to over 100 procedure codes within 11 families of codes. When 2 or more procedures within a family are performed on the same patient in a single session, the technical component (TC) of the highest priced procedure is paid at 100 percent; the TC of each subsequent procedure is paid at 75 percent. The reduction does not apply to the professional component.

The GAO estimates that considerable additional savings may be realized by expanding the MPPR to additional non-surgical, non-imaging procedures and by applying the MPPR to physician work, as well as to practice expense.

Page 2 – Barbara Pisaro Clark

GAO Recommendation

The Centers for Medicare & Medicaid Services should take further steps to ensure that fees for services paid under Medicare's physician fee schedule reflect efficiencies that occur when services are performed by the same physician to the same beneficiary on the same day.

CMS Response

We concur with GAO's recommendation. In the 2009 Physician Fee Schedule final rule (73 FR 69882) we indicated that we plan to perform a data analysis of non-surgical Current Procedural Terminology codes that are often billed together (e.g., 60-70 percent of the time) to determine whether there are efficiencies that would justify a payment reduction. We further indicated that we plan to review physician work as well as practice expense inputs. We agree that we should focus on code pairs that have the most impact on Medicare spending. We also agree that monitoring physician behavior will be necessary if the MPPR is expanded.

If reductions are warranted, we may propose either to expand the application of the MPPR or bundle additional services, as appropriate. Any proposed changes in our payment policy will be made through rulemaking and be subject to public comment.

In order to facilitate analysis of the issues raised by the GAO, we strongly urge GAO to include, as an appendix to this report, all the specific code pairs identified and used by the GAO in preparation of this report.

The Centers for Medicare & Medicaid Services appreciates GAO's analysis of the effects of expanding the MPPR, both in terms of the range of procedures and in applying it to physician work as well as to practice expense.

End Notes

[1] Medicare Part B covers physician and other outpatient services.

[2] On average, the physician work component accounts for about 52 percent of the total fee for each service, the practice expense component accounts for about 44 percent, and the malpractice component for about 4 percent.

[3] CMS also uses resource estimates for physician work and practice expenses to calculate indirect expenses—such as overhead, office equipment, and administrative staff salaries—for each service; thus, duplication of these resource estimates when services are commonly furnished together further contributes to excess payments.

[4] The seven contractors we interviewed together process claims in 28 states across the nation. CMS is in the process of integrating the administration of Medicare Part A (which covers hospital and other inpatient services) and Part B to new entities known as Medicare Administrative Contractors. The transition must be completed by October 2011.

[5] For this report, we will use "services commonly furnished together" to mean services performed by the same physician to the same beneficiary on the same day.

[6] We interviewed experts from the American College of Cardiology and American College of Radiology who had published articles on appropriate payments for Medicare physician services. We also interviewed an expert from the American Society of Interventional Radiology to understand how certain interventional radiology procedures are valued by the AMA-sponsored physician panels, since these procedures are commonly furnished on the same day with other services.

[7] Not all of the services included under the physician fee schedule are performed by physicians; some services (such as chemotherapy services or routine tests) may be performed by nurses or technicians.

[8] Primarily composed of physicians from the specialty societies, the Advisory Committee makes recommendations to the CPT Editorial Panel for either the creation of new codes or revisions to existing codes. The CPT Editorial Panel meets three times a year, and its actions can result in three outcomes: (1) a new or revised code is approved, (2) the proposal is postponed pending further information, or (3) the proposal is rejected.

[9] Estimates for physician work are developed by the RUC, while estimates for practice expenses are first reviewed by a subcommittee of the RUC—the Practice Expense Subcommittee, then submitted to the RUC for final recommendation to CMS.

[10] These phases are referred to as preservice, intraservice, and postservice. The RUC maintains a database that includes vignettes and physician work estimates for services that it has reviewed.

[11] Indirect expenses—overhead, administrative labor, and office expenses—are calculated by CMS in proportion to direct expenses and the physician work or clinical labor involved in providing each service.

[12] Medicare's physician payment system ranks services on a common scale based on the amount of resources needed to provide each service relative to a benchmark service—defined as a midlevel office visit. These relative resources are expressed as relative value units (RVU). (Thus, if a midlevel office visit has an RVU value of 1.0, a service with an RVU of 1.5 is estimated to be 50 percent more costly to provide.) RVUs for each service are converted into fees by adjusting them to reflect geographic differences in resource costs, then multiplying by a dollar conversion factor. For further details on the process CMS uses to set fees, see GAO, *Medicare Part B Imaging Services: Rapid Spending Growth and Shift to Physician Offices Indicate Need for CMS to Consider Additional Management Practices*, GAO-08-452 (Washington, D.C.: June 13, 2008), and *Medicare Physician Fees: Geographic Adjustment Indices Are Valid in Design, but Data and Methods Need Refinement,* GAO-05-119 (Washington, D.C.: Mar. 11, 2005).

[13] See 42 U.S.C. § 1395w-4(c)(2)(B)(i),(ii).

[14] Supplemental services are exempt from the MPPR.

[15] The MPPR applies only to the fee for the provision of the imaging test—generally performed by a technician. It does not apply to the fee for the interpretation of the imaging test—generally performed by a radiologist or other physician.

[16] Although the reduction is applied to the entire fee for each subsequent service, according to the rules we reviewed, the MPPR reflects duplication in practice expenses, not physician work. See 56 Fed. Reg. 59,502, 59,514-15 (Nov. 25, 1991); 62 Fed. Reg. 33,158, 33,171 (June 18, 1997); and 73 Fed. Reg. 69,726, 69,882 (Nov. 19, 2008).

[17] See 42 U.S.C. § 1395w-4(c)(2)(B)(ii).

[18] See 42 U.S.C. § 1395w-4(c)(2)(B)(v).

[19] The workgroup told us that it intends to review pairs that are performed together at a threshold below 90 percent after it completes review of the type A and B pairs.

[20] As of May 2009, specialty societies had recommended that each of the 22 type A and 31 type B service pairs be combined into single codes. The CPT Editorial Panel and the RUC have reviewed 25 of these proposals, and the RUC has forwarded its recommendations to CMS. CMS officials stated that they will publish these proposals and the agency's decisions in the proposed rule for 2010. (The proposed rule for 2010 was published on July 13, 2009.) The proposals on the remaining 28 service pairs are slated to be reviewed at upcoming CPT meetings.

[21] In addition to the workgroup's task of examining services commonly furnished together, the RUC is examining other misvalued services. For example, in June 2008, CMS forwarded a list of several hundred codes for its review. The list included codes in three different categories: (1) 114 services with the fastest growth, (2) 2,900 services with physician work estimates that had been developed over 20 years ago, and (3) over 320 services with rapid growth in practice expenses. The April 2009 RUC meeting agenda included over 2,000 pages of materials pertaining to these codes as well as other policies proposed by CMS.

[22] Estimates of excessive payments that were avoided for surgical services subject to the MPPR have not been available since this policy was implemented over 10 years ago.

[23] CMS recently expanded the imaging MPPR to include 10 additional services.

[24] MedPAC, *Report to the Congress: Medicare Payment Policy* (Washington, D.C.: 2006).

[25] CMS stated, in the 2009 final rule, that it will conduct data analysis and seek input from the RUC, MedPAC, and specialty societies to determine if an MPPR should be expanded to other (nonsurgical and nonimaging) services. See 73 Fed. Reg. 69,726, 69,882 (Nov. 19, 2008). Officials also told us that they expect to publish proposals for expanding the MPPR to other services in the proposed rule for 2010. (The proposed rule for 2010 was published on July 13, 2009.)

[26] Although the reduction is applied to the entire fee for each subsequent service, according to the rules we reviewed, the MPPR reflects duplication in practice expenses, not physician work. See 56 Fed. Reg. 59,502, 59,514-15 (Nov. 25, 1991); 62 Fed. Reg. 33,158, 33,171 (June 18, 1997); and 73 Fed. Reg. 69,726, 69,882 (Nov. 19, 2008).

[27] MedPAC, *Report to the Congress: Medicare Payment Policy.*

[28] Interventional radiology procedures generally include one or more surgical procedures that are accompanied by imaging services. While the surgical procedures are subject to the surgical MPPR, the imaging services are not. Physical therapy services are generally valued as 15-minute sessions. Officials from the AMA explained that time spent on preservice and postservice activities is spread across the number of services in a "typical" session to avoid duplication of practice expenses. However, we found that there was duplication of certain activities in the intraservice period. For example, time spent testing range of motion or muscle flexibility was duplicated in the physical therapy service pairs that we examined.

[29] We could not estimate savings from an MPPR for the physician work component of all service pairs because the RUC had not reviewed these services and the data required for this analysis were missing.

[30] AMA officials informed us that the RUC has recommended changes for this service pair that CMS could incorporate into the 2011 physician fee schedule.

[31] Experts we interviewed agreed that this methodology was a reasonable way of estimating efficiencies in physician work.

[32] The 5 Percent Standard Analytic File contains final action claims data submitted by noninstitutional providers, including physicians, physician assistants, clinical social workers, nurse practitioners, independent clinical laboratories, ambulance providers, and stand-alone ambulatory surgical centers.

[33] Thus, we excluded Part B services provided or ordered by physicians but paid under other fee schedules, such as prescription drugs, laboratory, and Durable Medical Equipment. We estimated that these services account for approximately one-third of total Medicare spending on physician-billed services.

[34] Certain services, including imaging tests, have two separate portions—a professional portion that represents the physician's interpretation of the test, and a technical portion that represents the actual performance of the test, generally by a technician. As such, the professional portion reflects the physician's work. We excluded services with a professional portion since CMS currently does not have policies in place to recognize efficiencies in physician work.

[35] These policies fell into three broad categories: (1) the National Correct Coding Initiative, which disallows payment for the second service because it is either a component of the first service or cannot reasonably be performed with the first service; (2) the global surgery payment policy, which generally disallows separate payment for certain services—such as evaluation and management—performed before and after a surgical service over a defined period of time, because reimbursement for these evaluation and management services is included in the surgical fee; and (3) the multiple procedure payment reduction (MPPR), which reduces payment for the second and subsequent services for certain surgical and imaging services. CMS officials we met with concurred that while they routinely issue payment policies on other individual services that are performed together, the three policies that we identified are the most comprehensive.

[36] We identified supplemental services as those listed in Appendix D: "Summary of CPT Add-on Codes" and Appendix E: "Summary of CPT Codes Exempt from Modifier 51", of the 2008 *AMA CPT Manual*.

[37] The total list of service pairs generated before any exclusions was approximately 165,000 pairs. After the exclusions, that number dropped to approximately 64,000. We then selected the top 350 service pairs that accounted for at least one-half of 1 percent of the total savings potential from the 64,000 service pairs.

[38] Preservice describes the activities involved prior to performing a specific procedure, such as obtaining a patient history; intraservice reflects the primary service performed, such as interpretation of an imaging test; and postservice includes activities performed following a procedure, such as signing a final report and discussing the findings with the referring physician.

[39] Physician time does not account for either the complexity and intensity of a procedure and the risk to the patient or the physician's skill required, but the time spent on activities in both the preservice and postservice phases is likely to be duplicated for procedures performed together by the same physician on the same patient on the same day.

[40] For example, if a service takes a total of 20 minutes, and the time spent on the preservice and postservice phases was 3 minutes and 2 minutes, respectively, the discount would be 25 percent.

In: Medicare Payment Policies and Issues ISBN: 978-1-61122-896-0
Editors: Alexander D. Hoffmann

Chapter 4

MEDICARE PROGRAM INTEGRITY: ACTIVITIES TO PROTECT MEDICARE FROM PAYMENT ERRORS, FRAUD, AND ABUSE

Holly Stockdale

SUMMARY

According to the 2009 Medicare Trustees report, total Medicare expenditures were $468 billion dollars in 2008 for 45 million beneficiaries. The Office of the Actuary projects overall Medicare spending to reach $507.1 billion for 2009. Because of a number of factors, such as advances in health care delivery and technology, an aging population, and overall increases in medical costs, spending on Medicare services is expected to grow more quickly than spending in the U.S. economy. As expenditures continue to rise in the nation's largest health insurance program, efforts to preserve the integrity of the program receive increased attention from policy makers.

In general, initiatives designed to fight fraud, waste, and abuse are considered program integrity activities. This includes processes directed at reducing payment errors as well as activities to prevent, detect, investigate, and ultimately prosecute health care fraud. As the agency responsible for administering Medicare, the Centers for Medicare and Medicaid Services (CMS) oversees a network of private contractors that perform various program integrity activities such as auditing providers, reviewing claims for medical necessity, and conducting investigations. Contractors develop and refer suspected cases of fraud to the Department of Health and Human Services Office of the Inspector General (HHS OIG) and the Department of Justice (DOJ) for further investigation and prosecution.

Medicare program integrity activities are funded in statute, largely through the Health Care Fraud and Abuse Control (HCFAC) and Medicare Integrity Programs (MIP), which were both established by the Health Insurance Portability and Accountability Act of 1996 (HIPAA, P.L. 104- 191). The HIPAA legislation provided CMS and federal law enforcement agencies with dedicated funds to coordinate Federal, state, and local activities to fight health care fraud. Beginning in FY2009, Congress approved additional discretionary funds to enhance these efforts.

This report provides an overview of Medicare's program integrity efforts. A description of key program integrity activities is presented as well as a discussion of the role that private contractors and law enforcement agencies play in maintaining Medicare's integrity. Detailed information on federal funding for program integrity efforts is also presented. The report concludes with a summary and analysis of recent efforts to oversee Medicare's program integrity activities.

INTRODUCTION

According to the 2009 Medicare Trustees report, total Medicare expenditures were $468 billion dollars in 2008 for 45 million beneficiaries.[1] The Office of the Actuary projects overall Medicare spending to reach $507.1 billion in 2009.[2] Because of a number of factors, such as advances in health care delivery and technology, an aging population, and overall increases in medical costs, spending on Medicare services is expected to grow more quickly than spending in the U.S. economy. As expenditures continue to rise in the nation's largest health insurance program, efforts to preserve the integrity of the program receive increased attention from policy makers.

As the agency responsible for administering Medicare, the Centers for Medicare and Medicaid (CMS) oversees a network of private contractors that conduct various program integrity activities. The six main types of activities are (1) conducting provider audits, (2) reviewing claims for medical necessity, (3) identifying and investigating fraud, (4) ensuring that Medicare pays only for services for which it has primary responsibility, (5) educating providers on Medicare billing procedures, and (6) identifying improper billing practices that affect both Medicare and Medicaid. Contractors refer suspected cases of fraud to the Department of Health and Human Services Office of the Inspector General (HHS OIG) and the Department of Justice (DOJ) for further investigation and prosecution.

Medicare program integrity activities are funded in statute, largely through the Health Care Fraud and Abuse Control (HCFAC) and Medicare Integrity Programs (MIP), which were both established by the Health Insurance Portability and Accountability Act of 1996 (HIPAA, P.L. 104- 191). The HIPAA legislation provided CMS and federal law enforcement agencies with dedicated funds to safeguard federal monies and prevent health care fraud, waste, and abuse.[3] Beginning in FY2009, Congress approved an additional discretionary investment of $198 million for FY2009 and $311 million for FY20 10 to further enhance Medicare's program integrity efforts.

This report provides an overview of Medicare's program integrity activities. The report begins with an introduction to the problem of health care fraud in Medicare. The report continues with descriptions of the types of program integrity activities undertaken by CMS to prevent fraud, waste, and abuse, and a discussion of the role that private contractors and federal law enforcement agencies play in maintaining Medicare's integrity. Detailed information on federal funding for anti-fraud efforts is also presented. The report concludes with a summary and analysis of recent efforts to oversee Medicare's program integrity activities.

Although this report addresses program integrity activities undertaken to prevent fraud in Medicare's private Part C and D programs, it is largely focused on Medicare's approaches to ensure integrity in its FFS program (Parts A and B), which constitute the largest share of Medicare spending.[4]

BACKGROUND ON MEDICARE

Medicare is the nation's health insurance program for persons aged 65 and older and certain disabled persons. Of the program's 45 million enrollees, approximately 85% are aged and the remaining 15% are disabled.[5] The majority of Medicare spending, nearly 75%, is for benefits provided by Parts A and B, the FFS portion of the program otherwise known as "original" or "traditional" Medicare. The remaining 25% is spent on private health care plans that deliver Medicare services to beneficiaries under Part C, the Medicare Advantage (MA) program, and Part D, the new prescription drug benefit.

Medicare consists of four distinct parts: Parts A, B, C, and D. Medicare Part A (Hospital Insurance) covers inpatient hospital, skilled nursing facility, home health, and hospice services. Medicare Part B (Supplementary Medical Insurance) covers a variety of other medical services, such as physician visits, outpatient hospital care, laboratory services, and durable medical equipment (DME)[6]. Beneficiaries also have the option to enroll in a private MA plan to receive all required Part A and B benefits, and a private Prescription Drug Plan (PDP) for prescription drug benefits. Most beneficiaries who opt to enroll in a private plan choose a MA-PD (Medicare Advantage Prescription Drug) plan for combined Part C and D coverage. Approximately 75% of beneficiaries receive services through original Medicare, and 25% receive services through a MA plan.

Medicare is administered by CMS within the Department of Health and Human Services. CMS contracts with private entities to oversee day-to-day operations and conduct program integrity activities for Parts A, B, C, and D. Each year, Medicare contractors process nearly 1.2 billion claims for over 1 million providers enrolled in the Medicare program. In addition to processing and paying claims, contractors conduct program integrity functions. Contractor activities are overseen by two departments within CMS: the Program Integrity Group and the Center for Drug and Health Plan Choice. The Program Integrity Group is responsible for oversight related to Parts A and B and the Center for Drug and Health Plan Choice is responsible for oversight activities related to Part C and D. On February 17, 2010, CMS announced the creation of a new Center for Program Integrity to oversee both Medicare and Medicaid program integrity activities.[7]

The Problem of Health Care Fraud

Renewed interest in health care reform has focused Congressional attention on the problem of health care fraud, waste, and abuse. Although the actual dollar value lost to health care fraud is unknown, fraud analysts and law enforcement officials estimate that anywhere between 3% and 10% of total health care expenditures are lost to fraud on an annual basis.[8] Not only does fraud and abuse contribute to the rising cost of health care, but it can also harm patients, particularly when medically necessary services are not provided or are provided unnecessarily.

Generally, the term "fraud and abuse" refers to misconduct in the delivery and financing of health care. Typically one thinks of financial misconduct when discussing health care fraud, however, delivering poor or substandard quality care has received increased attention from fraud enforcers in recent years.[9] Federal regulations define fraud and abuse separately. Specifically, Medicaid regulations define fraud as an intentional deception or misrepresentation made by a person with the knowledge that the deception could result in some unauthorized benefit to himself or some other person. Similarly, abuse is defined as provider practices that are inconsistent with sound fiscal, business, or medical practices, and result in an unnecessary cost to the Medicaid program, or in reimbursement for services that are not medically necessary or fail to meet professionally recognized standards for health care.[10] There is no corresponding definition of fraud and abuse in Medicare regulations.

Although health care fraud encompasses many different types of erroneous behavior, the types of fraud schemes being committed today share certain characteristics. According to law enforcement officials, fraud perpetrators often target public health insurance programs (Medicare and Medicaid) and private health plans simultaneously. Fraud schemes frequently span multiple states and can involve both providers of services, many of whom have little or no experience in health care, and beneficiaries. For example, in several recent cases, fraud perpetrators paid both providers and senior citizens kickbacks to obtain their billing numbers in order to submit fraudulent claims to Medicare. Other examples of recent fraudulent activity include billing for unnecessary services or tests provided to patients, submitting claims for services provided by unlicensed providers, and illegally marketing drugs or products for higher reimbursements.[11] Further, recent fraud investigations have revealed evidence of an increase in organized crime in health care. At a recent hearing before the House Energy and Commerce Health Subcommittee, the Inspector General of the Department of Health and Human Services (HHS) testified that health care fraud has become attractive to perpetrators of organized crime because the penalties are lower than for other organized crime-related offenses, there are low barriers to entry, fraud schemes are easily replicated, and a lack of data hampers detection efforts.[12]

Although there is some overlap, the types of fraud committed against Medicare's FFS program can be different than the types of fraud committed against Medicare's Part C and D plans. These differences stem largely from differences in Medicare's payment structure. In FFS, Medicare pays providers directly for a specified unit of service delivered to a beneficiary (i.e. procedure, visit, test, or group of services). This can create an incentive for providers to over-utilize health care services or provide more care to beneficiaries in order to maximize reimbursement. Examples of fraudulent activity in the FFS program include:

- Billing for services not furnished and/or supplies not provided.
- Altering claim forms, electronic claim records, medical documentation, etc., to obtain a higher payment amount (i.e. upcoding).
- Billing for services already provided (i.e. duplicate payments).
- Soliciting, offering, or receiving a kickback, bribe, or rebate, e.g., paying for a referral of patients in exchange for the ordering of diagnostic tests and other services or medical equipment.
- Billing non-covered or non-chargeable services as covered items.
- Billing separately for services or equipment included in global rate (i.e. unbundling).

In contrast, under Parts C and D, Medicare pays private health and PDP plans a fixed monthly payment amount per enrollee, otherwise known as capitation. The payment amount is made in advance for a pre-determined set of benefits, either Part A and B benefits administered by a MA plan or prescription drug benefits administered by a PDP plan. Under capitation, the monthly payment amount is fixed, regardless of the amount of services provided. Therefore, providers have an incentive to limit health services or provide fewer services to beneficiaries in order to maximize reimbursement. In Medicare Parts C and D, types of fraudulent activities may include:

- Engaging in fraudulent marketing practices (i.e. offering beneficiaries a cash payment to enroll, enrolling beneficiaries without their consent, conducting unsolicited door-to-door marketing, or using unlicensed agents).
- Selectively enrolling health enrollees (i.e. "cherry picking").
- Failing to provide medically necessary services.
- Inappropriately overestimating or underestimating bid amounts for payment.
- Imposing excessive beneficiary premiums.

Historically, Medicare's program integrity approaches have focused on combating fraud in the FFS sector. However, with enrollment in private Medicare plans on the rise and the addition of the new Part D drug benefit, program integrity approaches to fight fraud in capitated payment systems has become increasingly important.

Overview of Medicare Program Integrity

In Medicare, program integrity typically encompasses two types of activities: (1) processes directed at reducing payment errors or improper payments and (2) activities designed to prevent, detect, investigate, and ultimately prosecute fraud.

Since 1990, the Government Accountability Office (GAO) has declared Medicare at high risk for improper payments and fraud due to its size, scope, and decentralized administrative structure.[13] To protect the Medicare Trust Fund from improper payments, CMS contracts with private organizations to review claims to determine whether the services provided are medically reasonable and necessary. In Medicare, improper payments include both underpayments and overpayments to providers and largely result from provider billing mistakes or inadvertent claims processing errors. Although Medicare's claims review strategies do identify some instances of fraud, they are not specifically designed to do so. Of the claims that are reviewed, the majority are reviewed on a post-payment basis.

To protect the Medicare Trust Fund from fraud and abuse, CMS contracts with private organizations to conduct activities directed at identifying and detecting actual fraud. CMS typically classifies these functions as benefit integrity activities. Examples of benefit integrity methods include performing ongoing data analysis of claims to identify aberrant billing patterns, conducting fraud investigations, auditing providers, contacting Medicare beneficiaries and providers to verify that medical services were actually provided, and referring suspected cases of fraud to law enforcement personnel for prosecution. When these activities reveal suspected fraudulent activity, contractors develop and refer cases to the HHS OIG for further investigation and administrative sanctions. Fraud cases may then be referred to the DOJ for prosecution.

Types of Program Integrity Activities

To protect Medicare from improper payments, as well as fraud, waste, and abuse, Medicare contractors have historically conducted six main types of program integrity activities: cost report auditing, medical review, benefit integrity, Medicare secondary payer, provider education, and operating a

Medicare-Medicaid Data Match Program. These six functions are stipulated in law and are largely performed as part of CMS's MIP program. [14]

Cost Report Auditing

Part A Medicare providers such as hospitals, nursing homes, home health agencies, and other institutional providers are required to submit cost reports to CMS annually. [15] Cost reports contain information on the provider's allocation of costs across services. CMS contractors analyze these cost reports by conducting desk reviews. The objective of the desk review is to assess whether the reported costs are adequate and accurate, and to determine whether a more comprehensive, on- site audit is necessary. If the desk review reveals problems with the cost report, contractors may conduct field audits at the provider's place of business. Field audits are designed to ensure compliance with Medicare regulations and reimbursement policies and to obtain reasonable assurance that the cost report was prepared in accordance with Medicare laws, regulations, and instructions. The cost report auditing activity also includes audits of MA plan cost reports.[16] Part B providers (physicians, outpatient hospital, durable medical equipment providers, and others) are not required to submit cost reports to CMS.

Medical Review

Medical review activities are designed to identify and prevent payment errors and mistakes in billing. More specifically, medical review activities are conducted to ensure that a payment is appropriate for the service that is provided and meets professionally recognized standards of care. As part of this process, Medicare contractors review claims, largely through the use of automated computer edits, to verify that the services are (1) covered by Medicare, (2) provided by legitimate providers, (3) delivered to eligible beneficiaries, and (4) reasonable and medically necessary.[17] When an edit reveals a billing error or problem with a claim, contractors may conduct a manual pre-payment or post-payment claims review, request additional medical documentation from the provider, or contact beneficiaries to verify that the services were actually provided.[18]

Benefit Integrity

Benefit integrity involves the identification and investigation of potential fraud cases and referrals to law enforcement. CMS contractors hired to perform benefit integrity work may conduct national and regional data analysis to identify aberrant patterns of billing, request medical documentation from providers to verify services delivered, investigate beneficiary complaints related to fraud, and educate providers about fraud detection and prevention. When fraud is suspected, contractors refer cases to the OIG or law enforcement for further investigation, prosecution, or both. Benefit integrity activities may also include recoupment[19] of overpayments and suspension of future payments when fraud is suspected.

Medicare Secondary Payer (MSP)[20]

MSP activities ensure that Medicare pays only for those services where it has primary responsibility for payment. Under MSP rules, Medicare is prohibited from making payments for any item or service when payment has been made or can reasonably expect to be made by certain third-party payers. Statutorily, Medicare is the secondary payer to employer-based insurance plans, auto liability insurance, and workers compensation insurance. CMS maintains a comprehensive database of all Medicare beneficiaries' health insurance information and uses the database to conduct investigations related to MSP.

Provider Education

To help prevent errors and keep providers abreast of any changes in Medicare billing and coding procedures, contractors are required to conduct regular outreach and educational activities. Examples of educational activities include seminars, workshops, articles and fact sheets, and other website publications. Provider education activities also include developing resources for providers to help them avoid and detect fraud, waste, and abuse. When billing problems or improper payments are identified, CMS contractors are required to work with Medicare providers directly to correct mistakes.

Medicare-Medicaid Data Match Program

Referred to as the Medi-Medi program, this activity is designed to identify fraudulent or improper billing practices that affect both Medicare and Medicaid programs. By matching data across both programs, CMS investigates atypical billing patterns that may not be evident when analyzing the data from each program separately. When problems are identified, CMS works with the states to initiate payment recovery actions. CMS currently has Medi-Medi projects operating in 10 states.[21] According to HHS, in FY2008, 30 Medi-Medi cases were referred to law enforcement and over $27 million in overpayments were identified for collection. [22]

Types of Program Integrity Contractors

To conduct program integrity activities, Medicare contracts with an array of different contractors. The types of activities undertaken by these contractors vary depending on their Statement of Work (SOW). Some process and pay Medicare claims in addition to performing program integrity functions (i.e. Medicare Administrative Contractors or MACs). Others specialize solely in program integrity and fraud prevention activities such as Zone Program Integrity Contractors (ZPICs), Medicare Drug Integrity Contractors (MEDICs), Recovery Audit Contractors (RACs), the Comprehensive Error Rate Testing (CERT) contractor, and the Coordination of Benefits (COB) contractor. A brief description of each of these contractors and their scope of work are described below. This list is not exhaustive.

Medicare Administrative Contractors (MACs)

Congress, with the passage of the Medicare Prescription Drug, Improvement, and Modernization Act of 2003 (MMA, P.L. 108-173), mandated that the Secretary contract with MACs to process and pay Medicare claims.[23] Historically, fiscal intermediaries (FIs) performed claims administration functions for Part A providers (i.e. hospitals and facilities) and carriers performed claims administration functions for Part B providers (i.e. physicians). The MMA required that CMS replace the 40+ FIs and carriers with competitively selected MACs. In addition to processing and paying claims, these contractors perform select program integrity functions, including medical review of claims, identifying and recovering improper payments, conducting provider audits, educating providers on appropriate billing practices, and screening beneficiary complaints related to alleged fraud. The MMA required that CMS replace all FIs and carriers with MACs by October 2011. Currently, CMS has awarded all 19 MAC contracts – 15 to process claims for Part A and B providers (A/B MACs) and 4 to process claims for DME providers (DME MACs). As of January 2010, all 4 DME MACs and 9 A/B MACs were fully operational. The remaining six A/B MAC contracts are under procurement corrective action.

Program Safeguard Contractors (PSCs) and Zone Program Integrity Contractors (ZPICs)

Since 1997, Medicare has contracted with PSCs to detect and investigate potential fraud and abuse in Medicare's FFS program. CMS is in the process of transitioning these benefit integrity activities from PSCs to ZPICs. Once fully operational, ZPICs are expected to perform benefit integrity activities for Medicare Parts A, B, C, and D. Unlike CMS's contracting strategy for PSCs, there will not be separate ZPICs responsible for reviewing DME, home health, and hospice claims. Program integrity activities for all claim types will be conducted under a single ZPIC contract. ZPICs and PSCs conduct data analysis to identify improper billing patterns, perform provider audits, investigate fraud leads, refer cases to the OIG or DOJ for prosecution, and implement administrative actions to recover improper payments (i.e. pre-and post-payment claims review, payment suspension, payment denial, or recoupment of overpayments).

To facilitate coordination and communication among contractors, CMS established 7 ZPIC zones to align with the new MAC jurisdictions. The agency plans to have one ZPIC serving each zone. Five of these zones will encompass states identified by CMS as having high levels of fraudulent activity (California, Florida, Illinois, New York, and Texas). As of January 2010, CMS had awarded contracts for 4 ZPIC zones. The ZPICs operating in two of these zones are fully operational. The remaining two ZPIC awards were protested by other bidders.[24] Currently, the two ZPICs that are operational are performing anti-fraud activities in two of the five high-risk states – Florida and Texas.

Medicare Drug Integrity Contractors (MEDICs)

Medicare contracts with MEDICs to conduct program integrity activities in the Medicare prescription drug benefit program.[25] At the beginning of FY2009, CMS added fighting fraud, waste and abuse in Medicare Part C to the scope of work for the MEDICs. The MEDICs perform many similar functions as the ZPICs, including data analysis to identify patterns of erroneous billing, conducting investigations, referring cases to the OIG or DOJ for prosecution, and implementing administrative actions to recover improper payments. MEDICs are also responsible for auditing the fraud, waste, and abuse compliance programs that are a requirement for participation as a Part D plan in the Medicare program.[26] There are currently two regional MEDICs under contract to investigate fraud in the prescription drug program nationwide.[27]

Recovery Audit Contractors (RACs)

In 2003, Congress authorized a three year demonstration program in the MMA to test the use of a new type of administrative contractor in Medicare called a RAC. RACs are charged with identifying improper payments made in Part A and B Medicare and recouping overpayments. In 2006, Congress made the RAC program permanent and mandated its expansion nationwide by the year 2010.[28] On October 6, 2008, CMS announced the names of the four national RACs: Diversified Collection Services (DCS), CGI Technologies and Solutions (CGI), Connolly Consulting Associates, and Health Data Insights (HDI). Each RAC is responsible for reviewing claims for approximately one-fourth of the country. All providers who receive payment under Parts A and B could be subject to a RAC audit.[29] The statute does not authorize RACs to look for improper payments in the MA or PDP programs.

Although identifying potential fraud is not a RAC responsibility, the RACs are required to refer claims they believe may be fraudulent to CMS for further investigation. In February 2010, the OIG released a report indicating that during the three year demonstration program (2005 – 2008) RACs referred only two cases of potential fraud to CMS.[30]

Comprehensive Error Rate Testing (CERT) Contractor

CMS contracts with a CERT contractor to calculate improper payment rates for its FFS program.[31] In 2002, Congress enacted the Improper Payments Information Act (IPIA, P.L. 107- 300), which requires federal agencies to estimate and report an annual amount of improper payments for all programs and activities. The CERT contractor calculates three types of improper payment rates: 1) a national improper payment rate, 2) contractor-specific improper payment rates, and 3) improper payment rates by provider type. According to the agency, the contractor- specific improper payment rates are used to assess MACs, FIs, and carriers performance in paying claims accurately. The provider-specific rates are to see how well providers' are complying with Medicare's billing and coding requirements. On November 18, 2009, CMS reported a FY2009 national improper payment rate of 7.8%, or $24.1 billion in paid claims for original FFS Medicare. CMS produces midyear and annual improper payment reports, which can be accessed publicly on the agency website.[32]

National Supplier Clearinghouse (NSC) Contractor

The NSC is responsible for reviewing enrollment applications from DME suppliers and conducting site visits to confirm their compliance with Medicare enrollment standards (i.e. maintaining a physical facility and primary business telephone number). DME suppliers are required to re-enroll in Medicare once every three years in order to continue billing the program. The NSC conducts mandatory site visits upon initial enrollment and re-enrollment. The NSC may conduct random, unannounced site visits at other times if there is evidence that a supplier may be out of compliance. In the most recent (May 2009) Compendium of Unimplemented Recommendations, the OIG included a recommendation that CMS strengthen the DME supplier enrollment process by conducting more unannounced site visits.[33]

Coordination of Benefits (COB) Contractor

The main purpose of the COB contractor is to identify payments that are the responsibility of another or secondary payer. Statutorily, Medicare is the secondary payer to employer-based insurance plans, auto liability insurance, and workers compensation insurance. By using data match programs, the Medicare COB is responsible for the collection, management, and reporting of other health insurance coverage for Medicare beneficiaries. In January of 2001, the COB contractor assumed responsibility for researching and conducting all MSP claim investigations. There is one COB contractor that handles all program integrity functions related to MSP.

PROGRAM INTEGRITY PARTNERS

CMS shares responsibility for ensuring Medicare program integrity with the HHS OIG, the DOJ, and the Federal Bureau of Investigation (FBI). The OIG is an independent unit within HHS that has the primary responsibility for detecting health care fraud and abuse in all federal health care programs.[34] Most of its work, however, relates to the Medicare and Medicaid programs. The agency conducts audits of health care programs, providers, and agencies, and it performs criminal and civil investigations related to specific instances of health care fraud or abuse. CMS contractors, upon detecting potential fraud, will develop and refer cases to the OIG for further investigation and possible administrative sanctions.

The OIG has the authority to impose civil monetary penalties[35] and program exclusions[36] on Medicare providers that have been convicted of certain fraudulent activities. The OIG does not have the authority to prosecute offenders for violations of federal criminal law. In these instances, the OIG refers the case to the DOJ for prosecution. During FY2008, the OIG excluded a total of 3,129 individuals and entities from participating in Medicare, Medicaid, and other federal and state health care programs.[37]

The FBI is the lead investigative agency in the fight against health care fraud. Unlike the OIG, which has the authority to investigate fraud only in federal programs, the FBI has jurisdiction over both federal and private sector insurance programs. Typically, the agency investigates complex fraud schemes involving large-scale medical providers, such as hospitals and corporations. The FBI does not have the authority to impose sanctions. In FY2008, 2,434 FBI-led investigations resulted in 696 criminal health care fraud convictions.[38]

CMS contractors, the OIG, and the FBI all refer potential health care fraud cases to the DOJ for prosecution. Within the DOJ, the Civil and Criminal Divisions handle health care fraud. One of the enforcement tools for prosecuting health care fraud is the False Claims Act (FCA), which prohibits knowingly submitting false or fraudulent claims to the U.S. government. Lawsuits may be brought by private plaintiffs, known as relators or whistleblowers, under the FCA.[39] There are also 93 U.S. Attorneys Offices nationwide, which prosecute civil and criminal health care fraud. During FY2008, prosecutors for the DOJ and U.S. Attorneys Offices opened 957 new criminal and 843 new civil health care fraud investigations. This is compared to 878 new criminal and 776 new civil health care fraud investigations in FY2007.[40]

Finally, Medicare beneficiaries are a source for detecting fraud. Beneficiaries who suspect fraud can call the OIG's National Fraud Hotline at 1-800-HHS-TIPS. To educate beneficiaries on how to detect and report fraud and abuse, the Administration on Aging oversees Senior Medicare Patrol Projects, which recruit retired professionals in all 50 states to conduct one-on-one and group training sessions for Medicare beneficiaries.[41] Contractors investigating anomalies in billing patterns may also contact beneficiaries to verify that the services claimed were actually received by the beneficiary.

FUNDING FOR PROGRAM INTEGRITY ACTIVITIES

Medicare program integrity and anti-fraud activities are funded through the HCFAC and MIP programs. HCFAC and MIP were both established by HIPAA, which sought to increase and stabilize federal funding for health care anti-fraud activities. Specifically, HCFAC funds are directed to the enforcement and prosecution of health care fraud, whereas MIP funding supports the program integrity activities undertaken by CMS contractors. Prior to HIPAA, funding for Medicare's program integrity activities was taken from CMS's annual program management budget, which was subject to the appropriations process. This sometimes led to fluctuations in funding, as monies originally intended to support program integrity functions were redirected to fund ongoing Medicare operations, such as day-to-day claims processing functions. With the passage of HIPAA, HHS was ensured a stable funding source that it could commit to Medicare anti-fraud activities.[42]

HCFAC

Section 1128C of the SSA authorizes the establishment of the HCFAC program. The purpose of the program, which is jointly administered by the Secretary of HHS and the Attorney General, is to (1) coordinate federal, state, and local law enforcement efforts directed at controlling health care fraud and abuse; (2) conduct investigations, audits, evaluations, and inspections related to health care delivery and payment; (3) facilitate the enforcement of criminal and civil monetary penalties applicable to health care fraud; (4) provide for the establishment of safe harbors, advisory opinions, and fraud alerts; and (5) support the reporting and disclosure of adverse actions against health care providers. To fund the program, HIPAA established within the Hospital Insurance (HI) Trust Fund (Part A) an expenditure account called the HCFAC account. The HCFAC account funds the anti-fraud activities undertaken by HHS, DOJ, and the FBI. All amounts equal to monies collected from health care investigations and enforcement efforts are to be deposited into the HI Trust fund.[43]

MIP

Section 1893 of the SSA authorizes the establishment of the MIP program. Specifically, the authorizing language requires the Secretary to enter into contracts with eligible entities to conduct the following six activities: (1) medical review, (2) audits of cost reports, (3) determinations as to whether payment should not be, or should not have been, made by Medicare (otherwise known as Medicare Secondary Payer determinations), (4) education of providers of services, beneficiaries, and other persons with respect to payment integrity and benefit quality assurance issues, (5) developing and updating a list of items of DME, which are subject to prior authorization, and (6) the Medicare-Medicaid Data Match Program, or Medi-Medi program. **Table 1** shows HCFAC and MIP mandatory appropriations for selected fiscal years.

Discretionary Funding for Program Integrity Activities

Although CMS has requested additional discretionary funds to supplement the mandatory HCFAC appropriation since 2006, Congress didn't actually approve the adjustment until 2009. The FY2009 discretionary appropriation included $147 million for MIP, $19 million for the DOJ, $19 million for the OIG, and $13 million for CMS for a total of $198 million. For FY20 10 Congress approved an additional $311 million in discretionary funding for the HCFAC program, an increase of $113 million over the FY2009 level. The President's budget request for FY20 11 includes $561 million for Medicare and Medicaid program integrity activities, an increase of $250 million over the FY20 10 level. If approved, total funding for HCFAC in FY20 11 would amount to $1.7 billion. Table 2 shows HCFAC and MIP discretionary appropriations for FY2009- FY2011.

The President expects this additional discretionary investment for FY2011 to save approximately $9.9 billion over ten years (FY2011 – FY2021).[44] The budget request indicates that the agency plans to allocate $328.4 million of the $561 million to fighting fraud in Medicare, $47.7 million for program integrity activities in Medicaid, $90 million to the DOJ, and $94.8 million to the OIG. Approximately 50% of the $328.4 million for Medicare would be used to fund oversight activities in the MA and Part D programs. The remaining 50% would be directed towards expanding enforcement activities ($16.3M), increasing program oversight ($20.8M), implementing specific administrative and legislative proposals targeted towards fraudulent providers ($71.0M), funding regional fraud hotlines ($19.3M), conducting site visits to DME suppliers ($17.4M), expanding data analysis activities ($14.5M), and enhanced provider oversight efforts ($10.5M).[45]

Other Funding Sources for Program Integrity Activities

In addition to HCFAC and MIP mandatory funds, each year Congress appropriates discretionary funds to support overseeing and administering Medicare, Medicaid, and the Children's Health Insurance Program (CHIP). These monies are appropriated into CMS's program management account. For FY2010, Congress approved $3.5 billion for these activities, which include processing provider claims, paying the salaries of CMS staff, inspecting participating health care facilities, and conducting research and demonstrations. A portion of these funds are directed to program integrity functions.

Table 1. HCFAC and MIP Mandatory Appropriations for Selected Fiscal Years (1999-2011)

	1999	2001	2003	2005	2007	2009	2010	2011 (est)
HCFAC								
HHS	$8,273	$8,428	$31,143	$31,143	$31,746	$33,892	$33,892	$33,892
DOJ	$30,740	$43,469	$49,415	$49,415	$51,793	$55,328	$55,328	$55,328
OIG	$98,220	$130,000	$160,000	$160,000	$165,920	$177,205	$177,205	$177,205
FBI	$66,000	$88,000	$114,000	$114,000	$118,218	$126,258	$126,258	$126,258
MIP	$560,000	$680,000	$720,000	$720,000	$720,000	$720,000	$720,000	$720,000
Medi-	-	-	-	-	$24,000	$48,000	$60,000	$60,000
Medi								
TOTAL	**$763,233**	**$949,897**	**$1,074,558**	**$1,074,558**	**$1,111,677**	**$1,160,683**	**$1,172,683**	**$1,172,683**

Source: HCFAC Annual Reports for FY1999-FY2008, CMS Justification of Estimates for Appropriations Committees FY2003-FY20 11, and GAO Reviews of HCFAC Reports.

Table 2. HCFAC and MIP Discretionary Appropriations for FY2009 - FY20 11 (dollars in thousands)

	2009	2010	2011 (est)
HCFAC			
DOJ	$18,967	$29,790	$90,003
OIG	$18,967	$29,790	$94,830
CMS	$13,028	$31,100	$47,744
MIP	$147,038	$220,320	$328,423
TOTAL	**$198,000**	**$311,000**	**$561,000**

Source: CMS Justification of Estimates for Appropriations Committees FY2009-FY2011.

Oversight of Medicare's Program Integrity Efforts

There are a limited number of performance statistics and reports available to help policy makers evaluate the success of Medicare's program integrity efforts. Studies to date have generally examined the performance of the HCFAC and MIP programs separately. When the HIPAA legislation was passed in 1996, Congress mandated that DOJ and HHS report annually the results and accomplishments of its HCFAC efforts to the public. The legislation also requires that the GAO biennially assess the appropriateness and adequacy of HCFAC expenditures for fraud control efforts. However, Congress did not require that HHS, DOJ, or GAO evaluate the MIP program as part of these assessments. As a result, there is less empirical data available on MIP performance than on the results of the HCFAC program. To date, the most comprehensive evaluation on MIP program integrity efforts was a study released by GAO in September of 2006, which identified weaknesses in the methods CMS uses to allocate funds across five MIP program integrity activities (cost report auditing, medical review, benefit integrity, Medicare secondary payer, and provider education). This section summarizes findings from reviews and studies conducted on the HCFAC and MIP programs during the past decade.

Improper Payment Rates

When assessing the performance of the MIP program, CMS relies on statistics measuring the percentage of improper payments Medicare makes to providers each year. On November 18, 2009, CMS reported a FY2009 improper payment rate of 7.8%, or $24.1 billion in paid claims for original FFS Medicare. This is compared to a rate of 3.6% or $10.4 billion for FY2008. The agency attributes the increase between FY2008 and FY2009 to the application of stricter standards for reviewing claims.[46] At the same time CMS announced a calendar year 2007 improper payment rate of 15.4% or $12.0 billion for its MA program. This is compared to an improper payment rate of 10.6% or $6.8 billion for MA in 2006. An improper payment rate for Medicare Part D is under development.

Despite its value as a tool for estimating payment accuracy and administrative efficiency in claims processing, the improper payment rate does not measure fraud and abuse in the Medicare program. It is mainly a measure of administrative errors. The main types of payment errors in the FFS program are incorrect coding by providers, claims for medically unnecessary services, and claims submitted with insufficient or no documentation. According to the agency, the Part C payment error rate primarily reflects health plan errors in documenting members' diagnoses. **Table 3** lists the national paid claims error rates and the total in gross improper payments for selected years between 1996 and 2009.

HCFAC Annual Reports

HIPAA requires that every year HHS and the DOJ release a joint annual report to Congress on HCFAC results and accomplishments. Typically, these reports are released late summer or early fall and include numbers and examples of enforcement actions, program accomplishments, and amounts deposited into the HI Trust Fund resulting from health care fraud enforcement activities. Congress did not require that HHS and DOJ include expenditures or results for the MIP program in these reports. Therefore, they are only an indication of HCFAC's successes and challenges in the area of health care fraud enforcement and prosecution and not fraud prevention, which is a key objective of the MIP program. In addition, the authors do not separate out funding and expenditures for specific enforcement actions related to Medicare, Medicaid, or other federal health care programs.[48] The most recent annual HCFAC report released in November 2009 indicates that the federal government won or negotiated approximately $1.0 billion in judgments and settlements (fraud recoveries) during FY2008 and returned $1.94 billion to the HI Trust Fund (transfers).[49]

Figure 1 summarizes HCFAC fraud recoveries and transfers to the HI Trust Fund for fiscal years 1998 through 2008. The difference between the amount collected in fraud recoveries and the amount transferred to the HI Trust Fund in any given year can be attributed to the fact that fraud litigation is a lengthy process that can sometimes take several years. As a result, some of the judgments, settlements, and administrative actions won in one year may not result in monies being transferred to the trust fund until one or more years later.

Table 3. Medicare National Paid Claim Error Rates and Gross Improper Payments for Selected Years Between 1996 and 2009 (dollars in billions)

Year	National Paid Claims Error Rate (as a % of FFS expenditures)	Gross Improper Paymentsa
1996	14.2%	$23.2
1998	8.4%	$14.9
2000	9.4%	$16.4
2002	8.0%	$17.1
2004b	10.1%	$21.7
2006	4.4%	$10.8
2008	3.6%	$10.4
2009	7.8%	$24.1

Source: CMS and OIG Improper Payment Rate Reports for years 1996-2009.

a. CMS arrives at a gross improper payment amount by adding underpayments to overpayments.

b. From 1996-2002, the OIG calculated an error rate based on approximately 6,000 claims. Beginning in 2003, CMS took over the calculation of the error rate from OIG and expanded the sample of claims reviewed from 6,000 to approximately 128,000.

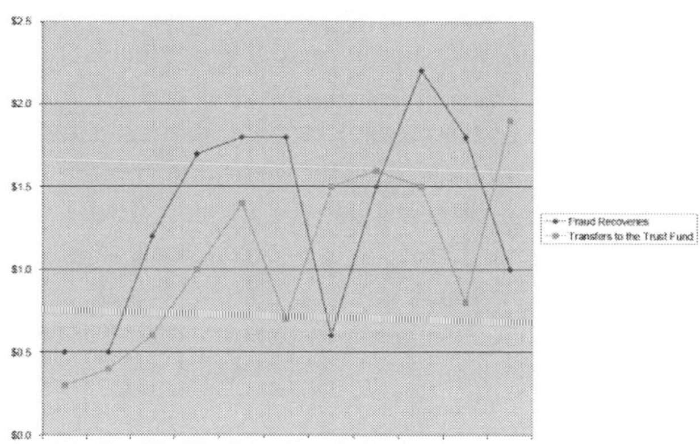

Source: HCFAC Annual Reports, FY1998-FY2008.

Figure 1. HCFAC Fraud Recoveries and Transfers to the Medicare HI Trust Fund for FY1 998- FY2008

Recoveries are amounts won or negotiated by the OIG and DOJ in any given year. They include criminal fines, civil monetary penalties, forfeitures, civil settlements and judgments. Recoveries vary annually depending on the number and types of fraud cases that are prosecuted. Between 1999 and 2003, recoveries steadily increased from \$0.5 to \$1.8 billion. Recoveries then dropped over \$1 billion between 2003 and 2004. Recoveries rose again from \$0.6 billion in 2004 to a high of \$2.2 billion in 2006. Recoveries have since dropped again to \$1.0 billion in 2008. The considerable increase in recoveries in 2006 can be attributed to a large settlement negotiated with Tenet Healthcare Corporation, operator of the nation's second largest hospital chain. Tenet agreed to pay the United States more than \$900 million over a four-year period for unlawful billing practices impacting the Medicare, Medicaid, and TRICARE programs.

Transfers are amounts collected resulting from HCFAC enforcement efforts. Between fiscal years 1998 and 2002, transfers to the Trust Fund steadily increased from \$0.3 billion dollars in 1998 to \$1.4 billion dollars in 2002. After a drop to \$0.7 billion in 2003, returns again increased between 2004 and 2006, holding relatively steady at approximately \$1.5 billion. Transfers again dropped in FY2007 to \$0.8 billion only to accelerate over \$1 billion dollars in FY2008 to \$1.94 billion – the largest amount collected over the program's ten year existence. According to the November 2009 HCFAC report, federal health care fraud enforcement activities have returned over \$13.1 billion dollars to the Medicare Trust Funds since 1997.

Table 4 shows the number of enforcement actions, including new criminal and civil health care fraud investigations and program exclusions for fiscal years 1999 through 2008. The number of new civil and criminal investigations has accelerated over the past ten years. However, there is debate as to whether this rise in enforcement actions is actually the result of more fraud and abuse in Medicare. Some experts contend that the increase is the result of having more resources to fight and detect illegal behavior, as opposed to an actual increase in the amount of fraud. Others note that the definition of what constitutes health care fraud has expanded over the years, making it appear as though fraud has escalated when the actual level has remained relatively steady.[50]

GAO HCFAC Reports

HIPAA also required that GAO submit a report to Congress every two years on HCFAC appropriations and deposits. Starting in June 1998, GAO released four reports using data from the HCFAC annual reports for years 1997 through 2003. The most recent and final report, released in April 2005, reviewed HCFAC activities for years 2002 and 2003.[51] Similar to the HCFAC annual reports, these studies do not include MIP in their analysis. In all four reports, GAO noted that while HCFAC deposit amounts reported to the HI Trust Fund were consistent with the HIPAA legislation, HHS included a measure of cost savings resulting from health care fraud enforcement efforts that could not entirely be attributed to the HCFAC program. [52] In addition, because fraud investigation and litigation can take several years, savings may not be realized until future years.

The Office of Management and Budget (OMB) echoed a similar finding in its Program Assessment Rating Tool (PART) evaluation of the HCFAC program in 2004 (see description below). Despite this weakness, GAO consistently found HHS and DOJ's accounting of HCFAC deposits and expenditures to be fiscally appropriate and accurate.

OMB Program Assessment Rating Tool (PART)[53]

In 2002, OMB evaluated the HCFAC and MIP programs separately using the PART, a 25- question survey addressing federal agency management and performance. The agency noted conflicting assessments for both programs. HCFAC received a "results not demonstrated" rating and criticized the OIG for not having sufficient performance measures to assess the program's progress in reducing fraud, waste, and abuse. Specifically, OMB noted that savings is not a good indicator of performance because it is too difficult to ascertain how much of the reported savings is the direct result of HCFAC activities conducted during the previous year.

Table 4. Summary of Health Care Fraud Enforcement Actions for FY1999-FY2008

	1999	2000	2001	2002	2003	2004	2005	2006	2007	2008
New Criminal Investigations	371	457	445	361	870	1,002	935	836	878	957
New Civil Investigations	91	233	188	221	231	868	778	915	776	843
Program Exclusions	2,976	3,350	3,746	3,448	3,275	3,293	3,804	3,422	3,308	3,129

Source: HCFAC Annual Reports, FY1 999-FY2008.

In contrast, the agency gave MIP an "effective" rating—the highest rating a program can receive. OMB attributes this largely to the OIG and CMS's measurement and reduction of the annual Medicare improper payment rate. CMS often cites the improper payment rate as a measure of its performance in protecting Medicare from fraud, waste, and abuse. In the PART report, OMB notes that at the time MIP was created in 1996, OIG estimated the improper payment rate at 14.2%. By 2006, the rate had dropped to 4.4% and by 2008 to 3.6%. However, as noted in Table 3, the Medicare improper payment rate rose to 7.8% in 2009.

Other GAO Reports

Subsequent GAO reports released over the last few years have raised questions about how HCFAC and MIP funding are being used. An April 2005 report on HCFAC funding for the FBI found that the agency could not adequately demonstrate that its share of HCFAC expenditures for FY2000-FY2003 were used for health care investigations. The study showed that funds previously devoted to fighting health care fraud at the FBI had been shifted to counterterrorism activities.[54]

In a report released in September 2006, the GAO identified weaknesses in CMS's approach for allocating MIP funds across the various program integrity activities (cost report auditing, medical review, benefit integrity, Medicare secondary payer, and provider education).[55] GAO noted that CMS bases its MIP allocation decisions on historical funding levels, as opposed to examining the relative effectiveness of one activity to another in ensuring Medicare program integrity. For example, despite receiving the largest share of MIP funds in FY2005, CMS has not yet developed a reliable quantitative measure to assess the impact of cost report audits of Part A providers on preventing fraud, waste, and abuse. GAO recommended that CMS develop additional methods for allocating MIP funds that take into account the effectiveness of MIP activities, as well as contractor performance, particularly in light of new vulnerabilities related to the prescription drug benefit.

OIG Audit and Evaluation Reports

Every year the OIG conducts audits, evaluations, and investigations of HHS programs. The recommendations that result from these assessments help lawmakers determine policies to improve the management and operations of these programs. In addition to individual audit and evaluation reports, the agency develops a number of annual reports synthesizing the outcomes of its work. For example, in its FY2009 Compendium of Unimplemented OIG recommendations, the agency identified the following priority recommendations for HHS to strengthen Medicare program integrity: implementing safeguards to prevent and detect fraud and abuse in Medicare Part D, ensuring DME Suppliers' compliance with Medicare standards, modifying payments to managed care organizations, improving CMS's performance evaluation process for PSCs, and improving oversight of hospices.[56] The OIG also produces an annual work plan describing the reviews and audits it plans to pursue in the coming year. For FY20 10, the agency plans to conduct over 100 studies and audits related to Medicare, the majority of which are related to Medicare Parts A and B.[57]

Concluding Observations

Program integrity activities encompass a broad set of strategies and processes designed to meet numerous objectives, including preventing improper payments, identifying and detecting fraud, investigating individuals suspected of committing Medicare fraud, and prosecuting offenders. To carry out the six main types of program integrity activities, CMS contracts with a number of different private organizations. The effectiveness of these efforts depends on close collaboration and coordination between CMS, its contractors, the OIG, and federal and state law enforcement agencies.

The implementation of HCFAC and MIP in 1996 provided CMS and Medicare enforcement agencies with a dedicated funding source to coordinate Federal, state, and local activities to fight health care fraud. From 1999 through 2009, resources available for program integrity and antifraud efforts increased from an estimated $0.8 billion in FY1999 to approximately $1.4 billion in FY2009, and the number of new civil and criminal fraud enforcement actions more than tripled. Furthermore, the amount of money transferred to the Medicare Trust Funds as a result of health care fraud enforcement activities has been steadily increasing. These statistics, however, do not apply to MIP activities, which receive the largest share of HCFAC funding. Recent GAO reports have raised questions about how MIP funding is being used and have recommended CMS develop more quantitative measures to assess the impact of MIP program integrity activities in the future.

Protecting Medicare from improper payments, fraud, and abuse is a complex and challenging undertaking for a number of reasons. To begin with, there are no reliable estimates on the actual amount of health care fraud, which makes it challenging for policy makers to determine the extent of resources needed to respond to the problem. Furthermore, fraud perpetrators are quick to adapt to investigative techniques and are continually devising more sophisticated schemes to defraud the system. Therefore, policymakers and administrators need to invest in a diverse mix of preventive and investigative program integrity methods to reduce Medicare's vulnerability to fraudulent activity. In recent years, fraud experts have urged CMS to adopt more preventive techniques to protect the program, such as increasing the volume of claims it reviews on a prepayment basis, applying stricter standards when reviewing provider enrollment applications, and conducting background checks on providers prior to allowing them to bill the Medicare program. In its FY2011 budget request, the agency indicates that it plans to direct at least $10.5 million in discretionary funding to conduct site visits and background checks of providers prior to enrollment.

As Medicare continues to grow in size and complexity, developing innovative strategies to ensure the integrity of the program become increasingly important. Both the House and Senate health care reform bills contain numerous provisions designed to strengthen Medicare's program integrity activities. For example, both bills would increase funding for the HCFAC program, introduce new penalties for fraudulent behavior, subject providers and suppliers to enhanced screening before allowing them to participate in Medicare, and require providers to establish compliance programs. The President's health reform proposal also includes provisions directed at reducing health care fraud, including requiring the establishment of a database to store information on health care fraud sanctions and modifying statutory requirements related to the pre-payment review of claims.

End Notes

[1] CMS Office of the Actuary, 2009 Medicare Board of Trustees Report, http://www.cms.hhs.gov/ReportsTrustFunds/downloads/tr2009.pdf.

[2] CMS Office of the Actuary, National Health Expenditures (NHE) Projections for 2009-20 19, http://www.cms.hhs.gov/NationalHealthExpendData/downloads/proj2009.pdf.

[3] Section 1128C of the Social Security Act (SSA) governs the Health Care Fraud and Abuse Control (HCFAC) program. Section 1893 of the SSA governs the Medicare Integrity Program (MIP).

[4] For additional information on oversight of the Part D benefit see CRS Report R40611, *Medicare Part D Prescription Drug Benefit*, by Patricia A. Davis.

[5] The disabled population includes persons under age 65 who receive cash disability benefits from Social Security or the Railroad Retirement systems for at least 24 months and persons under age 65 with end stage renal disease (ESRD).

[6] DME includes items such as hospital beds, wheelchairs, respirators, walkers, and artificial limbs specifically for home use.

[7] Currently, the Program Integrity Group is overseen by the CMS Office of Financial Management and the Medicaid Program Integrity Group by the Center for Medicare and Medicaid State Operations. For further information on the recent CMS reorganization visit: http://thehill.com/blogs/

[8] The National Health Care Anti-Fraud Association (NHCAA) estimates conservatively that 3% of all health care spending—or $68 billion—is lost to health care fraud. See NHCAA consumer alert available at: http://64.21 1.220. 122/eweb/DynamicPage.aspx?webcode=anti_fraud_resource_centr&wpscode=TheProblemOfHCFra ud. Also see the Federal Bureau of Investigation (FBI) Annual Financial Crimes Report available at: http://www.fbi.gov/publications/financial/fcs_report2008/financial_crime_2008.htm#health.

[9] Alice G. Gosfield, *Medicare and Medicaid Fraud and Abuse 2008 Edition*, pp. 5-6.

[10] 42 C.F.R. 455.2.

[11] *Department of Health and Human Services (HHS) and Department of Justice (DOJ) Annual Health Care Fraud and Abuse Control (HCFAC) Program Annual Report for FY2008*, September 2009, http://oig.hhs.gov/publications/docs/hcfac/hcfacreport2008.pdf.

[12] U.S. Congress, House Committee on Energy and Commerce, Subcommittee on Health, *Health Care Reform:Opportunities to Address Fraud, Waste, and Abuse*, Testimony of Daniel R. Levinson, HHS OIG, 111th Cong., June 25, 2009, *http://oig.hhs.gov/testimony/docs/2009/06252009_testimony_health_reform.pdf.*

[13] U.S. Government Accountability Office, *High Risk Series: An Update*, GAO-09-271, January 2009, http://www.gao.gov/new.items/d09271.pdf.

[14] Section 1893 of the SSA governs the MIP program. Other program integrity methods employed by CMS not discussed in this report include scrutinizing provider applications upon enrollment, conducting in-person site visits to provider locations to verify that they meet certain standards, and conducting inspections of provider facilities.

[15] Generally, Part A Medicare providers are paid under a prospective payment system (PPS). Under PPS, providers are paid pre-determined payment amounts based on specified units of service, such as hospital stays. When performing cost report audits, CMS reviews the few items that could affect a provider's payment under PPS, such as bad debt, organ procurement costs, payments for indirect and direct medical education, and the numbers of low-income patients hospitals serve. Recent studies conducted by GAO and MEDPAC have questioned the degree to which CMS's current audit process assesses the accuracy of Medicare costs for providers paid under PPS. See GAO-06-813, *Medicare Integrity Program: Agency Approach for Allocating Funds Should be Revised*, September 2006, http://www.gao.gov/ new.items/d068 13.pdf, and MEDPAC, *Report to the Congress: Sources of Financial Data on Medicare Providers*, June 2004, http://www.medpac.gov/publications/congressional_reports/june04_990_DataNeeds.pdf.

[16] Although the law requires that CMS annually audit the financial records of at least one-third of Part C MA plans, a GAO report released in July 2007 found that CMS did not document its process for ensuring that it met this requirement for years 2001-2005. See GAO-07-945, *Medicare Advantage: Required Audits of Limited Value*, July 2007, *http://www.gao.gov/new.items/d07945.pdf.*

[17] Computerized edits also check for errors such as incomplete or duplicate claims, claims where diagnosis codes do not match procedure codes, and unallowable code combinations.

[18] Manual pre-payment and post-payment claims reviews are initiated only after billing problems have been identified with a provider. Under pre-payment review, contractors will conduct a

manual medical review on a percentage of claims before payment is made. When conducting post payment review, contractors examine a statistically valid sample of paid claims from a provider. The majority of the claims that are reviewed are reviewed on a post-payment basis.

[19] Recoupment is recovering a Medicare overpayment by reducing present or future Medicare payments and applying the amount withheld against the debt.

[20] For more information on Medicare Secondary Payer, see CRS Report RL33587, *Medicare Secondary Payer - Coordination of Benefits*, by Hinda Chaikind.

[21] The Medi-Medi program is currently operating in the following 10 states: California, Texas, Washington, Pennsylvania, North Carolina, New Jersey, New York, Florida, Ohio, and Illinois. The Deficit Reduction Act of 2005 mandated the expansion of the Medi-Medi program nationwide. However, states receive no funding to participate in the program. In FY2010, the OIG plans to release a report on CMS's oversight and monitoring of the Medi-Medi program. See the OIG's FY2010 Workplan available at: http://www. oig.hhs. gov/publications/ docs/workplan/2010/Work_Plan_FY_2010.pdf.

[22] U.S. Congress, Senate Committee on the Judiciary, *Effective Strategies for Preventing Health Care Fraud*, Testimony of HHS Secretary William Corr, 111th Cong., October 28, 2009, http://www.hhs.gov/asl/testify/2009/10/t20091028a.html.

[23] Requiring the Secretary to contract with MACs was part of an overall legislative strategy to reform Medicare's administrative structure. Prior to the MMA, CMS was not authorized to select administrative contractors using a competitive selection process. Due to concerns that the enactment of Medicare would result in a large Federal intervention in the provision of health care, Section 1816 of the SSA authorized providers such as hospitals and nursing facilities to nominate their own FIs. Although the statute did afford the Secretary the authority to choose carriers to process Part B claims, Medicare regulations still limited the Secretary's flexibility in contracting. For example, the Secretary was prohibited from terminating an agreement with an administrative contractor without cause or the opportunity for a public hearing. Additionally, contracts were renewed automatically from year to year and were required to be cost-based and not performance-based. One goal of implementing the MAC initiative was to make Medicare contracting more consistent with the standard federal government contracting procedures governed by the Federal Acquisition Regulation (FAR). Today Section 1874A of the SSA requires that the Secretary use competitive procedures, which take into account quality as well as price, when selecting its claims processing contractors. The Secretary is also required to competitively select the MACs at a minimum once every 5 years and is authorized to include performance incentives in its contracts.

[24] CMS issued an RFP for ZPICs on May 1, 2008. On October 8th, 2008 CMS announced that it had awarded the first two ZPIC contracts to Health Integrity, LLC for Zone 4 (Texas, Oklahoma, Colorado, and New Mexico) and Safeguard Services, LLC for Zone 7 (Florida, Puerto Rico, and U.S. Virgin Islands). These two ZPICs are fully operational. In 2009, the agency awarded ZPIC contracts for Zone 5 (West Virginia, Virginia, North Carolina, South Carolina, Georgia, Alabama, Mississippi, Tennessee, Arkansas, and Louisiana) and Zone 2 (Alaska, Washington, Oregon, Montana, Idaho, Wyoming, Utah, Arizona, North Dakota, South Dakota, Nebraska, Kansas, Iowa, and Missouri) to AdvanceMed Corporation. Both of these awards to AdvanceMed were subsequently protested by other program integrity contractors. On January 25, 2010, the GAO upheld the protests for the Zone 2 and Zone 5 ZPIC contracts.

[25] For additional information on oversight of the Part D benefit see CRS Report R40611, *Medicare Part D Prescription Drug Benefit*, by Patricia A. Davis.

[26] According to a recent report released by the OIG, none of these audits were conducted by the MEDICs in FY2008. See OEI-03-08-00420, *Medicare Drug Integrity Contractors'Identification of Potential Part D Fraud and Abuse*, HHS OIG, October 2009, http://oig.hhs.gov/oei/reports/oei-03-08-00420.pdf. As a condition of participation in

Medicare, both MA and PDP plans are required to have in place a compliance plan which should include, among other elements, measures for detecting, correcting, and preventing fraud, waste, and abuse. Required elements of the plan include designation of a compliance officer; training, education, and effective lines of communication between the compliance officer and the organization's employees; procedures for ensuring prompt response to detected offenses; and procedures to voluntarily self-report potential fraud or misconduct to CMS (42 C.F.R 423.503 & 42 C.F.R 423.504).

[27] CMS awarded contracts to three regional MEDICs in FY2007. The three MEDIC contracts were consolidated into two in the Fall of 2008 when CMS did not renew the contract for one of the original three MEDICs.

[28] The legislation also provided CMS with the authority to pay RACs differently than other Medicare contractors, raising concerns among opponents of the RAC program. Historically, Medicare has paid its administrative contractors using cost-based contracts. Under a cost-based contract, Medicare reimburses contracting organizations for all necessary and proper costs incurred during the year. In contrast, the MMA legislation required Medicare pay RACs on a contingency basis. Under a contingency-based contract, contractors are reimbursed a portion, usually a percentage, from amounts recovered in improper payments. For additional information on Medicare's RAC program see CRS Report R40592, *Medicare's Recovery Audit Contractor (RAC) Program: Background and Issues*, by Holly Stockdale.

[29] This includes inpatient hospitals, physicians, skilled nursing facilities, inpatient rehabilitation facilities, DME suppliers, home health agencies, and other Part A or B providers.

[30] HHS OIG, *Recovery Audit Contractors'Fraud Referrals* , OEI-03-09-00130, February 2010, http://oig.hhs.gov/oei/reports/oei-03-09-00130.pdf.

[31] An improper payment is any payment that should not have been made or that was made in an incorrect amount. This includes duplicate payments, payments to ineligible recipients, payments for ineligible services, or payments for services not received. In Medicare, improper payments include both underpayments and overpayments to providers and largely result from provider billing mistakes and inadvertent claims processing errors.

[32] To access CMS annual improper payment rate reports see: https://www.cms.hhs.gov/ apps/ er_report/index.asp.

[33] HHS OIG, *Compendium of Unimplemented Recommendations*, May 2009, http://www. oig.hhs.gov/ publications/docs/compendium/compendium2009.pdf.

[34] For additional information on the authority, duties, and responsibilities of Inspectors General throughout the federal government see CRS Report 98-3 79, *Statutory Offices of Inspector General: Past and Present*, by Frederick M. Kaiser.

[35] Section 1128A of the SSA authorizes the Secretary to impose penalties and assessments on persons for engaging in certain activities. For example, a person who knowingly submits a false claim to a federal health care program is subject to a penalty of up to $11,000 for each item or service fraudulently claimed, an assessment of up to three times the amount fraudulently claimed, and possible exclusion.

[36] Section 1128 of the SSA authorizes the Secretary to exclude individuals and entities from participation in federal health care programs. Exclusions are authorized for convictions of criminal offenses related to the delivery of health care, including (1) Medicare or Medicaid fraud, (2) patient abuse or neglect, (3) felonies for other health care fraud, and (4) felonies for the illegal manufacture, distribution, prescription, or dispensing of controlled substances. The Secretary has discretionary authority to exclude individuals on other grounds, such as health care fraud offenses involving misdemeanors, license suspension or revocation, provision of unnecessary or substandard services, submission of false or fraudulent claims, and engaging in unlawful kickback arrangements.

[37] HCFAC Annual Report for 2008.

[38] HCFAC Annual Report for 2008.

[39] Under the Federal False Claims Act, 31 U.S.C. §§ 3729-3733, private citizens and relators may file suit on behalf of the U.S. government. Relators are private persons with direct knowledge of health care fraud who file complaints on behalf of the federal government. They are entitled to a percentage of any fraud recoveries.

[40] HCFAC Annual Report for 2008.

[41] The OIG collects annual performance data on these projects and its most recent report can be accessed at:*http://www.smpresource.org/Content/NavigationMenu/ResourcesforSMPs/OIG Reports/May09OIGPerformanceReport* .pdf .

[42] In addition, historically, Medicare relied heavily on "pay and chase" methods, which entailed paying claims and then chasing after providers to recover inappropriate payments. Long-term financial support was intended to assist CMS in developing more innovative and preventive strategies to combat fraud and abuse, such as reviewing claims prior to payment as opposed to after payment.

[43] As specified in Section 1817(k)(C) of the SSA, amounts equal to the following are to be deposited into the Federal Hospital Insurance Trust Fund from the U.S. Treasury: (1) amounts equaling unconditional gifts and bequests; (2) criminal fines recovered in cases involving a federal health care offense as defined in Title 18 U.S.C. § 982(a)(6)(B); (3) civil monetary penalties and assessments imposed in health care cases, including amounts recovered under titles XI, XVIII, and XIX, of the SSA and Chapter 38 of Title 31 of the U.S.C.; (4) amounts resulting from the forfeiture of property by reason of a federal health care offense; and (5) penalties and damages obtained under the False Claims Act, 31 U.S.C. §§ 3729-3933.

[44] Department of Health and Human Services Budget in Brief for 2011, p.2, http://www.hhs.gov/asrt/ob/docbudget/2011budgetinbrief.pdf.

[45] *CMS Justification of Estimates for Appropriations Committees Fiscal Year 2011*, pp. 161-178, http://www.cms.hhs.gov/PerformanceBudget/Downloads/CMSFY11CJ.pdf.

[46] See CMS Press Release dated November 18, 2009, available at: [H:\CMS Administration\ Improper Payments\HOW NEW STANDARDS FOR TOUGHER ERROR RATE WERE APPLIED IN THIS YEARS 2009 IMPROPER PAYMENTS REPORT.mht. Prior to 2008, Medicare's Quality Improvement Organizations (QIO) were responsible for calculating the error rate for inpatient hospitals. The improper payment rate for all other FFS claims was calculated by the agency's CERT contractor. Beginning in 2009, the agency transferred the responsibility for calculating the improper payment rate for inpatient hospitals from the QIOs to the CERT contractor. According to the agency, at least one reason for the increase in the FFS error rates between 2008 and 2009 was that the QIOs were using different claims review processes and a different measurement methodology to calculate the amount of improper payments. Now that the CERT contractor is responsible for reviewing all FFS claims, the review procedures for inpatient hospital claims are consistent with the review procedures applied to all other FFS claims.

[47] GAO-06-581T, *Challenges Continue in Meeting Requirements of the Improper Payments Information Act*, April 2006, http://www.gao.gov/new.items/d06581t.pdf.

[48] The HIPAA legislation does not require that HHS or DOJ separately track Medicare and non-Medicare expenditures. DOJ officials commented in a 2002 GAO Report on the HCFAC program that it is not practical to separate non- Medicare and Medicare expenditures because of the nature of health care fraud (GAO-02-73 1: Medicare, Health Care Fraud and Abuse Control Program for Fiscal Years 2000 and 2001, June 2002). Health care fraud cases typically cross several health care programs, making it difficult to attribute expenses and recoveries to separate programs.

[49] HCFAC Annual Report for 2008.

[50] Health Care Fraud and Abuse: Practical Perspectives, Chapter 4, 2004.

[51] GAO-05-134, *Health Care Fraud and Abuse Control Program: Results of Review of Annual Reports for Fiscal Years 2002 and 2003*, April 2005, http://www.gao.gov/new.items/d05134.pdf.

[52] The OIG defines cost savings as funds put to better use as a result of implemented legislative or other program initiatives.

[53] See Office of Management and Budget Program Assessment Rating Tool website at http://www.whitehouse.gov/omb/rewrite/part/index.html for PART assessments of the MIP and HCFAC programs.

[54] GAO-05-388, *Federal Bureau of Investigation: Accountability over the HIPAA Funding of Health Care Investigations is Inadequate*, April 2005, *http://www.gao.gov/ new.items/d05388.pdf.*

[55] GAO-06-8 13, *Medicare Integrity Program, Agency Approach for Allocating Funds Should be Revised, September 2006*, http://www.gao.gov/new.items/d06813.pdf.

[56] The OIG Compendium of Unimplemented Office of Inspector General Recommendations can be accessed at: http://www.oig.hhs.gov/publications/compendium.asp.

[57] The annual OIG Work Plan can be accessed at: http://www.oig.hhs.gov/ publications/ workplan.asp.

In: Medicare Payment Policies and Issues ISBN: 978-1-61122-896-0
Editors: Alexander D. Hoffmann

Chapter 5

MEDICARE'S RECOVERY AUDIT CONTRACTOR (RAC) PROGRAM: BACKGROUND AND ISSUES

Holly Stockdale

SUMMARY

Recovery Audit Contractors, or RACs, are private organizations that contract with the Centers for Medicare and Medicaid Services (CMS) to identify and collect improper payments made in Medicare's fee-for-service (FFS) program. CMS projects improper FFS payments to amount to approximately $10.4 billion or 3.6% of all paid Medicare claims in 2008. Congress originally required the Secretary of the Department of Health and Human Services to conduct a three-year demonstration program using RACs in the Medicare Prescription Drug, Improvement, and Modernization Act of 2003 (MMA, P.L. 108-173). In December 2006, Congress passed the Tax Relief and Health Care Act of 2006 (TRHCA, P.L. 109-432), which made the program permanent and mandated the expansion of RACs nationwide by 2010. CMS began the national rollout of the permanent program in 19 states in March 2009.

CMS initiated the RAC demonstration in March 2005 in three states—California, Florida, and New York. After a preliminary status report revealed that the three participating RACs had returned $54.1 million to the Medicare

Trust Funds during its first year of operation, CMS expanded the demonstration to two additional states—Massachusetts and South Carolina. The agency concluded the pilot in March 2008. According to the final evaluation of the demonstration, the RACs returned $693.6 million in overpayments to the Medicare Trust Funds over the course of three years.

Throughout the demonstration, CMS continuously highlighted the success of the RAC initiative in protecting the fiscal integrity of Medicare. However, the demonstration and subsequent permanent program have raised concerns among policymakers and industry groups because Medicare pays RACs differently than it pays other administrative contractors. Historically, Medicare's administrative contractors have been paid a fixed annual budget for a defined scope of work. In contrast, Congress mandated that CMS pay RACs using contingency fees. A contingency fee is a negotiated payment, typically a percentage, for every overpayment recovered. Under a contingency fee payment system, contractors receive no additional administrative funding. This type of compensation has been criticized for incentivizing RACs to aggressively audit and deny provider claims.

This report provides an overview of the RAC program along with a brief history of improper payments in Medicare. A description of the medical review processes used by RACs and how it compares with other Medicare administrative contractors is also presented. The report concludes with a discussion of current issues. This report will be updated as needed.

Background on Medicare

Medicare, authorized under Title XVIII of the Social Security Act, is the nation's health insurance program for persons aged 65 and older and certain disabled persons.[1] In 2008, Medicare expenditures totaled approximately $468 billion for 45 million beneficiaries.[2]

Medicare consists of four distinct parts: Parts A, B, C, and D. Medicare Part A (Hospital Insurance) covers inpatient hospital services, skilled nursing facility services, home health, and hospice services. Medicare Part B (Supplementary Medical Insurance) covers a variety of other medical services, such as physician visits, outpatient hospital care, laboratory services, and durable medical equipment. Parts A and B constitute the fee-for-service (FFS) portion of the program, otherwise known as "original" or "traditional" Medicare. Beneficiaries also have the option to enroll in a private Part C or

Medicare Advantage (MA) plan to receive Part A and B benefits, and a private Part D or Prescription Drug Plan (PDP) for drug coverage.

The agency responsible for administering Medicare is the Centers for Medicare and Medicaid Services (CMS) at the Department of Health and Human Services (HHS). CMS contracts with a variety of private entities to carry out the day-to-day operations of the program, such as paying provider claims, detecting alleged fraud and abuse, and overseeing the quality of care delivered to beneficiaries.[3] As opposed to specializing in one particular function, these entities are often responsible for performing multiple administrative activities under one contract. For example, in addition to processing claims, Medicare's administrative contractors may enroll providers in the Medicare program, educate physicians on appropriate billing practices, adjudicate appeals, and identify and recover improper payments.

Brief Introduction to Improper Payments

An improper payment is any payment that should not have been made or that was made in an incorrect amount. This includes duplicate payments, payments to ineligible recipients, payments for ineligible services, or payments for services not received. In Medicare, improper payments include both underpayments and overpayments to providers and largely result from provider billing mistakes and inadvertent claims processing errors.[4]

Since 1990, the Government Accountability Office (GAO) has declared Medicare at high risk for improper payments and fraud due to its size, scope, and decentralized administrative structure.[5] In 2002, Congress enacted the Improper Payments Information Act (IPIA, P.L. 107-300), which requires federal agencies to estimate and report an annual amount of improper payments for all programs and activities.[6] HHS began estimating an error rate for its Medicare FFS program in 1996. At that time, improper payments totaled an estimated $23.2 billion dollars, or 14.2% of total paid claims. That same year, Congress passed the Health Insurance Portability and Accountability Act (HIPAA, P.L. 104-191), which included provisions designed to increase and stabilize funding for activities directed at reducing health care fraud and improper payments in federal health programs. In addition to creating a Health Care Fraud and Abuse Control (HCFAC) program, HIPAA established the Medicare Integrity Program, or MIP, to decrease improper payments in Medicare.[7] Since 1996, the improper payment rate has progressively declined, reaching $10.8 billion, or 3.9% of total paid claims in 2007.[8]

RECOVERY AUDIT CONTRACTORS (RACS) IN MEDICARE

In the Medicare Prescription Drug, Improvement, and Modernization Act of 2003 (MMA, P.L. 108-173) Congress authorized a demonstration project for recovery audit contractors (RACs) in Parts A and B of the Medicare program. Recovery auditing is the term used to describe activities directed at identifying and recovering overpayments.[9] The legislation required that the Secretary enter into contracts with RACs for the purpose of identifying Medicare overpayments and underpayments, and recouping overpayments for services for which payment is made under Parts A and B.[10] The legislation also granted CMS the authority to reimburse RACs using contingency fees. A contingency fee is a negotiated payment, typically a percentage, of every overpayment recovered. CMS conducted the demonstration in five states (California, Florida, Massachusetts, New York, and South Carolina) between March 2005 and March 2008. Over the course of three years, the RACs returned $693.6 million in overpayments to the Medicare Trust Funds and corrected a total of $1 billion in improper payments (overpayments and underpayments) at a cost of only 20 cents for every dollar collected, a return of 5 to 1.[11]

Table 1. States Covered by Each RAC Contractor

Region	Contractor	States
A	Diversified Collection Services (DCS) with subcontractor PRG Shultz	Maine, Massachusetts, New Hampshire, New York, Rhode Island, Vermont
B	CGI Technologies and Solutions with subcontractor PRG Shultz	Michigan, Indiana, Minnesota
C	Connolly Consulting Associates with subcontractor Viant Payment Systems	Colorado, Florida, New Mexico, and South Carolina
D	Health Data Insights with subcontractor PRG Shultz	Arizona, Montana, North Dakota,

Source: CMS Website on RACs. Available at http://www.cms.hhs.gov/RAC/.

Prior to the conclusion of the demonstration, Congress passed the Tax Relief and Health Care Act of 2006 (TRHCA, P.L. 109-432), which made RACs permanent and mandated their expansion nationwide by January 1, 2010. The legislation was passed in December 2006; one month after a preliminary status report on the demonstration was released. [12] The statutory language expanding the RAC program required rather than authorized the Secretary to reimburse RACs using contingency fees. The legislation also granted the Secretary permission to pay RACs for identifying underpayments. Additional requirements include stipulations related to deposits of overpayments, audit and recovery periods, contractor qualifications, and a mandate for an annual performance report.[13] As in the demonstration, RACs are not authorized to look for improper payments in the MA or PDP programs.

On October 6, 2008, CMS announced the national rollout of the permanent program and released the names of the four RAC contractors: Diversified Collection Services (DCS), CGI Technologies, Connolly Consulting Associates, and Health DataInsights (HDI).[14] Beginning in March 2009, the four RACs began reviewing claims for select states in approximately one-fourth of the country. More states will be added to each RAC's jurisdiction as the program expands over the next two years.[15] All providers who receive payment under Medicare Parts A and B are subject to a RAC audit, including inpatient hospitals, physicians, skilled nursing facilities, inpatient rehabilitation facilities, DME suppliers, home health agencies, and other Part A or B providers.

The RACs were to begin conducting outreach for the permanent program in November 2008. However, shortly after announcing the names of the four new RACs, CMS imposed an automatic stay on the implementation of the nationwide program after two unsuccessful bidders for a RAC contract—Viant Payment Systems and PRG Schultz—filed a protest with the GAO. Viant and PRG, which served as RACs in the demonstration program, have subsequently settled their protest with the agency and are now acting as subcontractors for the permanent RACs. **Table 1** lists the regions and initial 19 states served by each of the four RAC contractors.

Claims Review Process Used by RACs

To identify improper payments, RACs are instructed to use a combination of both automated and complex review processes.[16] Under automated review, there is no human review of the claim or medical record. Computer edits within the claims processing system automatically check claims for evidence of improper coding or mistakes. RACs may use automated review only when the following two conditions are met: (1) there is certainty that the service is not covered by Medicare, and (2) there exists a written Medicare policy, such as a Medicare statutory provision, regulation, national or local coverage determination,[17] or manual instruction that specifies the circumstances under which a service will not be covered by Medicare. RACs may also use Medicare articles or coding guidelines approved by CMS to serve as the basis for an automated review.

In the absence of written Medicare policy, RACs are required to perform complex review. Complex review involves human review of the medical record and other documentation supporting the claim. RACs must use complex review in situations where there is a high probability that the claim contains an overpayment. They are also instructed to refer to appropriate medical literature and clinical judgment when making complex claim determinations. Although there is no specific requirement that RACs consult with physicians when conducting complex review, CMS does mandate that RACs use nurses and certified coders to review all medical records. All Medicare administrative contractors, including RACs, are required to employ one full-time medical director to oversee the claims review process. Although this was not a requirement for the RACs during the demonstration program, it has been mandated for the permanent program.

To select claims for review, RACs utilize data analysis. Although the actual data analysis techniques used by the contractors is proprietary, the process typically involves examining billing histories of providers to identify unusual or suspicious claims and comparing billing patterns to peers in a provider group to identify aberrancies. RAC contractors are also encouraged to review reports prepared by the HHS Office of Inspector General (OIG) and the GAO to identify claims likely to contain improper payments.

Comparison of Claims Review Processes between RACs and other Medicare Administrative Contractors

There are other contractors that review Medicare claims for improper payments as part of their administrative responsibilities. These include

Medicare Administrative Contractors (MACs), Fiscal Intermediaries (FIs), and Carriers;[18] Medicare's Comprehensive Error Rate Testing, or CERT, contractor; Program Safeguard and Zone Program Integrity Contractors (PSCs and ZPICs); and Quality Improvement Organizations or QIOs.[19] All of these contractors have the authority to review any claim they suspect may be improper, subject to certain limitations. An improper payment determination may be made for claims that were incorrectly coded, claims for services that were not medically necessary, claims resulting from incorrect payment amounts, and claims for services that were already provided (duplicate claims).

Although the claims review processes followed by RACs is relatively similar to that of other Medicare contractors, there are some differences. For example, MACs, FIs, Carriers, PSCs, and ZPICs can review claims prior to payment, otherwise known as pre-payment review. RACs, the CERT contractor, and QIOs can only review claims post-payment.

Table 2. Comparison of Medicare Contractors' Claims Review Processes

	RAC	MAC, FI, Carrier	CERT	PSC, ZPIC	QIO
When claims can be selected for review	Post-payment	Pre-payment and post-payment	Post-payment	Pre-payment and post-payment	Post-payment
Claim look-back period	Up to three years; not before October 1, 2007	Up to four years	Up to four years	Up to four years	Up to four years
Medical Director	Required	Required	Required	Required	Required
Staffing requirements for claims review	Nurses, therapists, and certified coders	Nurses and therapists; physician consultants and other health professionals in the various specialties as needed	Nurses and therapists; physician consultants and other health professionals in the various specialties as needed	Nurses and therapists; physician consultants and other health professionals in the various specialties as needed	Nurses and therapists; physician consultants and other health professionals in the various specialties as needed

Source: CRS Analysis of CMS Manual Instructions, RAC SOW, and CMS documentation related to Medicare's claims review programs.

Additionally, the statute and CMS have set restrictions on how many years contractors can "look- back" and select claims for review. These time periods are called "look-back" periods. Unless there is evidence of fraud, Medicare regulations prohibit contractors from reviewing claims more than four years past the date the claim was initially paid. During the demonstration program, the RACs were authorized to review claims in accordance with this four-year look-back period. However, in response to concerns from providers that RAC requests for medical records were becoming too burdensome, CMS reduced the claim look-back period from four to three years in the permanent program. Medicare's other administrative contractors will still be allowed to look- back four years. In the permanent program, RACs will also be prohibited from reviewing any claim paid prior to October 1, 2007.

Finally, CMS manual instructions direct certain administrative contractors to use physician consultants and other health professionals in the various specialties as necessary to perform complex review of medical documentation. This is not a requirement for RACs. **Table 2** highlights the similarities and differences among the various contractor claims review processes.

CONCERNS RELATED TO THE RAC PROGRAM

Payment

The RAC legislation provided CMS with the authority to pay RACs differently than it pays other administrative contractors. Historically, Medicare has paid its contractors using cost-based contracts. Under a cost-based contract, Medicare reimburses organizations for all necessary and proper costs incurred during the year. In contrast, the MMA legislation required that the Secretary pay RACs on a contingency basis. Under a contingency-based contract, contractors are paid a percentage of every overpayment they identify and collect from the provider. [20] They receive no additional funding as part of the contract.

This is the first time a contingency fee reimbursement mechanism has been used in the Medicare program to pay a contractor. CMS would not release data on the fees paid to each RAC during the demonstration program, asserting that the information was proprietary and therefore not disclosable. However, the agency did decide to make public the contingency percentages for each of the four permanent RACs, which range from 9.0% to 12.5% for each contractor.[21] According to CMS, RAC contracts were competitively awarded to the organization that met the agency's technical standards, such as knowledge of Medicare billing and coverage policies, and bid the lowest contingency percentage for a particular region.[22]

Opponents of the program charge that paying contractors on a contingent basis creates an incentive for RACs to aggressively audit and deny claims. Provider groups such as the American Hospital Association (AHA) and the American Medical Association (AMA) have requested that CMS remove the contingency fee payment structure and compensate RACs as they do other Medicare contractors—by paying them a fixed annual amount for a defined scope of work.[23] This concern was magnified during the demonstration program because participating RACs were allowed to retain their contingency fees even if their overpayment determinations were overturned on appeal. CMS subsequently changed this in the permanent program. RACs are now required to return contingency fees for all overpayment determinations overturned on appeal.

Opponents also assert that a contingency fee compensation mechanism encourages RACs to inaccurately or inappropriately deny claims. In May 2007, a California House Delegation led by Representative Lois Capps and Deven Nunes wrote to CMS indicating that Inpatient Rehabilitation Facilities (IRFs) in California were reporting nearly universal denial rates associated with admissions for joint replacement procedures during the RAC demonstration.[24] In response, CMS hired an independent validation contractor to re-review a sample of the RAC's determinations. After the independent validation contractor disagreed with the RAC's denials in 40% of the cases, CMS directed the RAC to stop its review of IRF claims in California.[25] On November 7, 2007, Representative Lois Capps introduced the Medicare Recovery Audit Contractor Program Moratorium of 2007 legislation (H.R. 4105), which would have placed a one- year moratorium on the implementation of the RAC program. The bill was referred to the House Committee on Energy and Commerce and the Committee on Ways and Means but did not become law.

In response to provider concerns, CMS will be requiring all RACs to request permission before beginning an audit related to a particular payment issue. The agency has also hired a RAC validation contractor to perform accuracy reviews on a sample of randomly selected overpayments identified by each RAC.[26] At a minimum, this audit would be performed annually. The results of the accuracy audit would not directly affect the RAC contingency fees but would be one of the performance metrics used to evaluate the RAC's effectiveness.

Trust Fund Recoveries

Throughout the three-year demonstration, RACs returned $693.6 million to the Medicare Trust Funds and corrected more than $1.03 billion in improper payments.[27] Provider groups claim that this overstates the actual net savings to the Trust Funds. At the time the final RAC evaluation was released there were still appeals pending, which were not accounted for in the final numbers. The appeals process can take months to years, depending on the provider's willingness to appeal to higher levels, meaning that funds initially recouped and returned to the Trust Funds may then have to be paid back to the provider. Further, provider groups assert that providers that do appeal an overpayment determination are often successful.

Table 3. Provider Appeals of RAC Overpayments

	Total # of Overpayments	# of Overpayments Appealed at any Level	% of Overpayments Appealed at any Level	# of Appeals Decided in Provider's Favor	% of Appeals Decided in Provider's Favor	Total % of Over payments Decided in Provider's Favor
3-Year Evaluation *(as of 3/27/08)*	525,133	73,266	14%	24,376	33.3%	4.6%
September 2008 Appeals Update *(as of 6/30/08)*	525,133	102,705	19.6%	35,819	34.9%	6.8%
January 2009 Appeals Update *(as of 8/31/08)*	525,133	118,051	22.5%	40,155	34.0%	7.6%

Source: The Medicare Recovery Audit Contractor (RAC) Program: An Evaluation of the 3-Year Demonstration released in June 2008 and Updates to the Evaluation of the RAC Program released in September 2008 and January 2009.

The final evaluation of the RAC demonstration indicates that providers appealed 14% of the total number of overpayment determinations made by the RACs (525,133 out of 1,167.9 million reviewed claims). Out of the overpayments that were appealed, 33% were overturned in the provider's favor. CMS has since updated the evaluation report with more recent appeals statistics.[28] As of August 31, 2008, providers chose to appeal 22.5% of the total number of overpayment determinations made by the RACs, up from 14% at the conclusion of the demonstration. The percentage of appealed claims decided in the provider's favor rose slightly from 33% to 34%. Additionally, out of the total number of appeals, the percentage overturned and decided in the provider's favor increased from 4.6% to 7.6%. The agency plans to release a final report with updated numbers on the total dollar value returned to the Trust Funds in the coming months.

Recoupment

Medicare regulations grant the Secretary the authority to recoup overpayments made to Medicare providers.[29] In 2003, Congress set limitations on the Secretary's authority to recoup overpayments with Section 935 of the MMA. Prior to the MMA, Medicare had the authority to recoup an overpayment regardless of whether or not the provider had elected to appeal the overpayment determination. Medicare would then repay the overpayment if the provider was successful in his or her appeal. Section 935 of the MMA restricts the Secretary from recouping overpayments, if an appeal has been initiated, until a decision has been made at the second level of the appeals process. CMS manual instructions, however, require that providers wishing to delay or prevent recoupment of an overpayment file a valid appeal within 30 days from the date they receive an overpayment demand letter.[30] If they do not file an appeal within 30 days, CMS reserves the right to initiate recoupment on day 41 after the demand letter is sent. CMS contends that while Medicare providers still have the statutorily mandated 120 days to file a first level appeal, the Secretary maintains the authority to begin recouping those funds prior to the 120 days.[31] However, at any time during those 120 days if a provider files an appeal, the Secretary must stop recoupment proceedings.

Certain providers assert that CMS's requirement that providers file an appeal within 30 days of the initial overpayment determination to delay recoupment is in conflict with Section 935 of the MMA. In July 2008, over 30 hospitals in South Carolina filed a complaint against the Secretary alleging that CMS had unlawfully recouped $30 million in alleged overpayments identified during a RAC audit. The hospitals claim that CMS recouped these overpayments prior to their receiving a decision at the second level of the appeals process. According to the complaint, the hospitals did not receive an overpayment demand letter from the RAC in time to issue a valid appeal and stay recoupment proceedings. The hospitals also contend that Section 935 of the MMA precludes recoupment entirely until a provider has an opportunity to appeal at both the first and second levels of the appeals process. In September 2006, CMS published a proposed rule implementing the limitation on recoupment. Two years later, in September 2008, CMS issued a change request detailing instructions for the rule's final implementation.[32]

Provider Burden

After identifying claims likely to contain improper payments, RACs may request medical records from the provider to substantiate a claim. During the demonstration, provider groups maintained that RAC audits were onerous to providers, sometimes requiring they respond to multiple medical record requests over the course of several weeks. In addition to copying and sending medical records to the RAC, providers must also complete the paperwork to initiate an appeal if they disagreed with the RAC's determination. Providers assert that RAC audits are time-consuming and take providers away from patient care. They are particularly burdensome for single practitioners or small group practices that sometimes have to close their offices to respond to an audit request.

CMS has made certain changes to the permanent program that may alleviate some of these concerns. For example, during the demonstration, RACs were allowed to set their own limits on medical record requests. In October 2008, CMS released the maximum number of records RACs can request in 2009. The limits range from 10-50 medical records in a 45-day time period for certain physician types to 10% of the average claims paid per month for inpatient hospitals, skilled nursing facilities, inpatient rehabilitation facilities, and hospices (up to a maximum of 200) per 45 days.[33] Although the limits are smaller for smaller provider types, certain practitioners remain concerned because the limits apply to each provider's National Provider Identifier (NPI). The NPI is a unique provider billing number that applies to all health care providers. Because some providers, particularly facilities such as hospitals, have multiple NPIs the medical record requests could continue to be administratively burdensome. CMS intends to further clarify its medical record policy related to facilities with multiple NPIs in the coming months.

Upcoming Evaluations

On July 11, 2008, John Dingell, Chairman of the House Energy and Commerce Committee; Charles Rangel, Chairman of the House Ways and Means Committee; Pete Stark, Chairman of the House Ways and Means Subcommittee on Health; Frank Pallone, Chairman of the House Energy and Commerce Subcommittee on Health; and Representative Lois Capps wrote a letter to the GAO requesting that the agency undertake a study of the RAC program. As part of its study, the GAO will be examining any actions CMS is taking to prevent future improper payments in high-risk areas identified during the demonstration as well as the agency's plans for the ongoing monitoring and oversight of its RAC contractors. The OIG is also conducting a study of the RAC initiative, which is expected to be completed in March 2010.

Concluding Observations

Improper payments pose a significant risk to Medicare. In FY2010, Medicare spending is expected to exceed $500 billion for approximately 47 million elderly and disabled beneficiaries.[34] Excluding improper payments in the Part C and D programs, overpayments in Medicare FFS amount to over $10 billion annually.

Historically, CMS has relied on its claims administration contractors to reduce improper payments in the Medicare program. However, shortly after HHS began reporting the first Medicare improper payment rate in 1996, concerns surrounding the contractors' effectiveness at safeguarding the program began to emerge. As noted by various experts, at least one contributing factor to the perceived weakness in this area was budget constraints and the lack of incentives for contractors to direct specific efforts at reducing payment errors.[35] Prior to the MMA, which mandated contracting reform, Medicare statute precluded CMS from offering financial incentives to its contractors to improve performance. Contractors were paid under cost-based contracts, which prohibited them from making a profit. Additionally, these entities were evaluated based on their ability to pay claims quickly and efficiently and not necessarily accurately. Therefore the RAC program, which authorizes the use of payment incentives to reimburse contractors, could be viewed as an opportunity for CMS to enhance its program integrity efforts.

On the other hand, paying contractors a fee for every improper payment they identify and recover has many policymakers and provider groups concerned. Results from the demonstration showed that while the RACs were successful in returning millions of dollars to the Medicare Trust Funds, some of their audits were inaccurate and overly burdensome for providers, raising questions about CMS's oversight of the program. The agency has since made a number of changes to the permanent program to mitigate some of these concerns, such as requiring RACs to return all contingency fees for overpayments overturned on appeal, hiring a validation contractor to review RAC audits, and setting limits on the number of medical records RACs can request from providers at one time. However, anxiety among providers remains. As the roll-out of the permanent program unfolds, results of the upcoming GAO and OIG evaluations will likely be critical to helping policymakers assess the pros and cons of using recovery audit contractors in Medicare.

ACKNOWLEDGMENTS

Sibyl Tilson, Patricia Davis, and Hinda Chaikind contributed to this report.

End Notes

[1] Of the program's 44 million enrollees, approximately 85% are aged and the remaining 15% are disabled. For an overview of the Medicare program, see CRS Report RL33712, *Medicare: A Primer*, by Hinda Chaikind.

[2] Centers for Medicare and Medicaid Services (CMS) Office of the Actuary, *2009 Medicare Trustees Report*. Available at http://www.cms.hhs.gov/ReportsTrustFunds/downloads/tr2009.pdf.

[3] For additional information on Medicare contractors' and their varied responsibilities see CRS Report RL34217, *Medicare Program Integrity: Activities to Protect Medicare from Payment Errors, Fraud, and Abuse*, by Holly Stockdale.

[4] Although improper payments may be fraudulent, they are not meant to be a measure of fraud. Generally, fraud involves intentional acts of deception or representation to deceive with knowledge that the action or representation could result in gain.

[5] U.S. Government Accountability Office, *High-Risk Series: An Update*, GAO- 09-271, January 2009, p. 5, http://www.gao.gov/new.items/d09271.pdf.

[6] The law requires agencies to annually identify programs and activities vulnerable to significant improper payments, estimate the amount of overpayments or underpayments, and report to Congress on steps being taken to reduce such payments. For additional information on the Improper Payment Act see CRS Report RS22587, *Improper Payments Information Act of 2002: A Brief Introduction*, by Virginia A. McMurtry and Garrett Hatch.

[7] For additional information on Medicare's anti-fraud activities, including HCFAC and MIP, see CRS Report RL34217, *Medicare Program Integrity: Activities to Protect Medicare from Payment Errors, Fraud, and Abuse*, by Holly Stockdale.

[8] Between 1996 and 2002, the HHS Office of the Inspector General (OIG) was responsible for calculating Medicare's improper payment rate. In 2003, CMS took over this responsibility. Over the years the adequacy and accuracy of CMS's calculation of Medicare's improper payment rate has been questioned by the GAO and OIG. In 2006, the GAO reported that reductions in the improper payment rate could not be attributed to improved payment controls, but instead were the result of changes CMS had made to its methodology for calculating the improper payment rate. See GAO Report, GAO-07-92, *Agencies' Fiscal Year 2005 Reporting under the Improper Payments Information Act Remains Incomplete*, November 2006, http://www.gao.gov/new.items/d0792.pdf. Most recently, the OIG reported problems with the agency's calculation of the FY2006 and FY2008 improper payment rates for Durable Medical Equipment (DME). In a report released on May 12, 2009, an independent OIG audit of CMS's DME error rate revealed a significantly higher error rate than the rate calculated by CMS. See HHS OIG Report, A-01-09-00500, *Independent Contractor's Review of DME Claims from the FY 2008 Comprehensive Error Rate Testing Program*, May 2009, http://www.oig.hhs.gov/oas/reports/region1/10900500.pdf.

[9] In 2003, in a memorandum to the heads of executive departments and agencies, the Office of Management and Budget (OMB) defined a recovery audit as a review and analysis of an agency's books, supporting documents, and other available information that is designed to identify overpayments to contractors due to payment errors. See OMB Memo, *Programs to Identify and Recover Erroneous Payments to Contractors, M-03-07*, January 16, 2003, http://georgewbush-whitehouse.archives.gov/omb/memoranda/m03-07.html.

[10] Recoupment is recovering a Medicare overpayment by reducing present or future Medicare payments and applying the amount withheld against the debt.

[11] U.S. Congress, House Committee on Small Business, Subcommittee on Regulations, Health Care, and Trade, *The Impact of CMS Regulations and Programs on Small Healthcare Providers*, Testimony of Tim Hill, Director of Office of Financial Management, CMS, 111th Cong., 2nd sess., May 14, 2008.

[12] The first report released in November 2006 indicated that RACs operating in California, Florida, and New York returned $54.1 million to the Medicare Trust Funds in year one (FY2006). Subsequent status reports indicated returning $247.4M in year two of the demonstration (FY2007) and $693.6 million over the course of the three-year demonstration (March 2005-March 2008). All status reports can be accessed on the CMS website at http://www.cms.hhs.gov/RAC/02_ExpansionStrategy.asp.

[13] The statute requires that the Secretary retain a portion of amounts recovered in its program management account to support the activities of the recovery audit contractor program. Remaining recoveries are to be applied to reduce expenditures under parts A and B.

[14] CMS, "CMS Announces New Recovery Audit Contractors to Help Identify Improper Medicare Payments," press release, October 6, 2008, http://www.cms.hhs.gov/apps/media

[15] For a map of the states included in each region visit the CMS website at http://www.cms.hhs.gov/RAC/Downloads/ Four%20RAC%20Jurisdictions.pdf.

[16] The following types of claim determinations may be considered improper by a RAC: (1) claims that were incorrectly coded, (2) claims resulting from incorrect payment amounts, (3) claims for services that do not meet Medicare's coverage criteria (i.e., services that are considered medically unnecessary), and (4) claims for services that were already provided

(duplicate claims). Final Request for Proposal (RFP) or Statement of Work (SOW) for Recovery Audit Contractors. RFP-CMS-2007-0022. Amended version dated November 7, 2007. Available on CMS website at http://www.cms.hhs.gov/RAC/01_Overview.asp#TopOfPage.

[17] Medicare makes coverage decisions at the national and local level. National Coverage Determinations or NCDs are national policy statements issued by the central office which grant, limit, or exclude Medicare coverage for a specific medical service, procedure, or device. Local Coverage Determinations or LCDs are coverage decisions made at the local level by Medicare's claims administration contractors. LCDs are only binding on a contractor's local service area. The majority of Medicare's coverage determinations are made at the local level.

[18] MACs process claims for Part A and B providers, FIs process claims for Part A providers, and Carriers process claims for Part B providers. In the Medicare Prescription Drug, Improvement, and Modernization Act (MMA, P.L. 108-173), Congress required the Secretary to reform its administrative contracting procedures. CMS refers to these legislatively mandated changes as contracting reform. Under contracting reform, the agency is gradually replacing the 40+ FIs and Carriers with 19 MACs. As of January 2009, CMS had awarded all 19 MAC contracts for participation in the Medicare program.

[19] MACs, FIs, and Carriers process and pay provider claims. Medicare's CERT contractor is responsible for measuring and reporting Medicare's improper payment rate. PSCs and ZPICs are Medicare's anti-fraud contractors, and QIOs monitor the quality of care delivered to beneficiaries. As of August 1, 2008, QIOs are no longer responsible for reviewing inpatient hospital claims. This responsibility has now been transferred to MACs and FIs. However, the QIOs will remain responsible for performing quality of care reviews, hospital-requested higher-weighted DRG reviews, reviewing beneficiary appeals, and EMTALA (anti-dumping) reviews. For additional information on Medicare contractors' and their varied responsibilities see CRS Report RL34217, *Medicare Program Integrity: Activities to Protect Medicare from Payment Errors, Fraud, and Abuse*, by Holly Stockdale.

[20] RACs are also paid a fee for every underpayment they identify and return to providers.

[21] See CMS Website on Recent Updates on the RAC program for the agency's announcement on the RAC contingency fees: http://www.cms.hhs.gov/RAC/03_RecentUpdates.asp.

[22] Individual communication with Division of Recovery Audit Operations at CMS, and RAC Request for Proposals (RFP). Amendment #3. RFP-CMS-2007-0022. November 28, 2007. Accessible at FedBizOpps.Gov website: https://www.fbo.gov/index?s=opportunity&mode=form&id=5c8c7d4b00249ba579d4d77d64bd0aea&tab=core&_cvie w=1.

[23] Letter to Chairman Rangel, Chairman Stark, Representative Capps, and Representative Nunes from the American Hospital Association (AHA), California Hospital Association, and Healthcare Association of New York State. December 10, 2007; and testimony of the American Medical Association (AMA). May 14, 2008. House Small Business Committee Subcommittee on Regulations, Healthcare, and Trade. Hearing. The Impact of CMS Regulations and Programs on Small Healthcare Providers.

[24] A copy of the letter and press release can be accessed on Congresswoman Lois Capp's website at http:/www.house.gov/list/speech

[25] PRG-Shultz, the subcontractor to three of the four RACs selected to participate in the demonstration program, was the RAC for California in the demonstration program.

[26] See CMS Website on Recent Updates on the RAC program: http://www.cms.hhs.gov/RAC/03_RecentUpdates.asp.

[27] CMS, *The Medicare Recovery Audit Contractor (RAC) Program: An Evaluation of the 3-Year Demonstration*, June 2008, http://www.cms.hhs.gov/RAC/Downloads/ RAC%20Evaluation%20Report.pdf. This is the final net savings after accounting for approximately $40 million paid in underpayments, the total costs to operate the RAC program ($201.3M), and $46 million returned to providers on appeal, and $14 million in re-review of IRF claims.

[28] See Updates to the Evaluation of the 3-Year RAC Demonstration. September 2008 and January 2009. Available at http://www.cms.hhs.gov/RAC/02_ExpansionStrategy.asp#TopOfPage.

[29] 42 CFR 405.371

[30] CMS. Medicare Financial Management Manual. Chapter 3 - Overpayments. http://www. cms. hhs.gov/manuals/ downloads/fin106c03.pdf.

[31] In accordance with Section 1869 of the SSA, providers wishing to contest an overpayment determination have 120 days from the date of the initial determination on a claim to file an appeal.

[32] See CMS Proposed Rule, 71 FR 55404, and September 22, 2006. Limitation on Recoupment of Provider and Supplier Overpayments. The change request can be accessed at http://www.cms.hhs.gov/Transmittals/downloads/ R141FM.pdf.

[33] For more detailed information on the Medical Record Limits for RACs see the following CMS Fact Sheet: http://www.cms.hhs.gov/RAC/Downloads/RAC%20 Medical%20Record%20 Request%20Limits.pdf.

[34] DHHS, Fiscal Year 2010, Budget in Brief, May 7, 2009. Available at http://www.hhs. gov/asrt/ob/ docbudget/ 2010budgetinbrief.pdf.

[35] David A. Hyman, "HIPAA and Health Care Fraud: An Empirical Perspective," *CATO Journal*, Spring/Summer 2002, pp. 151-178. Thomas H. Stanton, "Fraud-And-Abuse Enforcement in Medicare: Finding Middle Ground," *Health Affairs*, July/August 2001, pp. 28-42. GAO-01-817, Medicare Management: CMS Faces Challenges to Sustain Progress and Address Weaknesses, p. 21. Available at http://www.gao.gov/new.items/d01817.pdf.

CHAPTER SOURCES

The following chapters have been previously published:

Chapter 1 – This is an edited, reformatted and augmented version of Congressional Research Service publication, Report RL30526, dated August 18, 2010.

Chapter 2 – This is an edited, reformatted and augmented version of Congressional Research Service publication, Report R40907, dated August 6, 2010.

Chapter 3 – This is an edited, reformatted and augmented version of United States Government Accountability Office publication GAO-09-647, dated July 2009.

Chapter 4 – This is an edited, reformatted and augmented version of Congressional Research Service publication, Report RL34217, dated March 15, 2010.

Chapter 5 – This is an edited, reformatted and augmented version of Congressional Research Service publication, Report R40592, dated May 21, 2009.

INDEX

A

B

C

F

G

H

I

J

K

L

M